100 Questions & Answers About Restless Legs Syndrome

Sudhansu Chokroverty, MD, FRCP, FACP

Professor and Co-Chair of Neurology
Program Director of Clinical Neurophysiology & Sleep Medicine
New Jersey Neuroscience Institute at JFK Medical Center
Seton Hall University
Edison, NJ

DISCARD
FCPL discards materials that are outdated
and in poor condition. In order to make
room for current, in-demand materials,
underused materials are offered for
public sale

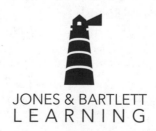

JONES & BARTLETT
L E A R N I N G

World Headquarters

Jones & Bartlett Learning
40 Tall Pine Drive
Sudbury, MA 01776
978-443-5000
info@jblearning.com
www.jblearning.com

Jones & Bartlett Learning
Canada
6339 Ormindale Way
Mississauga, Ontario L5V 1J2
Canada

Jones & Bartlett Learning
International
Barb House, Barb Mews
London W6 7PA
United Kingdom

Jones & Bartlett Learning books and products are available through most bookstores and online booksellers. To contact Jones & Bartlett Learning directly, call 800-832-0034, fax 978-443-8000, or visit our website, www.jblearning.com.

Substantial discounts on bulk quantities of Jones & Bartlett Learning publications are available to corporations, professional associations, and other qualified organizations. For details and specific discount information, contact the special sales department at Jones & Bartlett Learning via the above contact information or send an email to specialsales@jblearning.com.

Copyright © 2011 by Jones & Bartlett Learning, LLC

All rights reserved. No part of the material protected by this copyright may be reproduced or utilized in any form, electronic or mechanical, including photocopying, recording, or by any information storage and retrieval system, without written permission from the copyright owner.

The author, editor, and publisher have made every effort to provide accurate information. However, they are not responsible for errors, omissions, or for any outcomes related to the use of the contents of this book and take no responsibility for the use of the products and procedures described. Treatments and side effects described in this book may not be applicable to all people; likewise, some people may require a dose or experience a side effect that is not described herein. Drugs and medical devices are discussed that may have limited availability controlled by the Food and Drug Administration (FDA) for use only in a research study or clinical trial. Research, clinical practice, and government regulations often change the accepted standard in this field. When consideration is being given to use of any drug in the clinical setting, the healthcare provider or reader is responsible for determining FDA status of the drug, reading the package insert, and reviewing prescribing information for the most up-to-date recommendations on dose, precautions, and contraindications, and determining the appropriate usage for the product. This is especially important in the case of drugs that are new or seldom used.

Production Credits

Executive Publisher: Christopher Davis
Editorial Assistant: Sara Cameron
Associate Production Editor: Leah Corrigan
Associate Marketing Manager: Katie Hennessy
Manufacturing and Inventory Control
  Supervisor: Amy Bacus
Composition: Glyph International

Cover Design: Carolyn Downer
Cover Images: (top) © Dmitriy Shironosov/
  ShutterStock, Inc., (bottom left)
  © Les3photo8/Dreamstime.com,
  (bottom right) © Photos.com
Printing and Binding: Malloy, Inc.
Cover Printing: Malloy, Inc.

Library of Congress Cataloging-in-Publication Data
Chokroverty, Sudhansu.
  100 questions and answers about restless legs syndrome (RLS) / S. Chokroverty.
    p. cm.—(100 questions and answers)
  title: Hundred questions and answers about restless legs syndrome (RLS)
  Includes index.
  ISBN 978-0-7637-8094-4 (alk. paper)
  1. Restless legs syndrome—Miscellanea. 2. Restless legs syndrome—Popular works. I. Title.
  II. Title: Hundred questions and answers about restless legs syndrome (RLS).
  RC548.5.C46 2011
  616.8'498—dc22
                                                        2010025890

6048

Printed in the United States of America
14 13 12 11 10   10 9 8 7 6 5 4 3 2 1

Contents

The stigma of restless legs syndrome (RLS) as a psychosomatic disorder that began in the late 19th- and early 20th-century writings of Wittmack, Beard, and Oppenheim still lingers on in the 21st century in the minds of many people not adequately educated in the topic. We still see headlines like "RLS is a fabrication of the greedy pharmaceutical companies to invest in a 'disease mongering' entity." These headlines totally ignore the scientific evidence based on many sophisticated investigations, including genome-wide association studies, which strengthened the biological basis of RLS. These skeptics should simply ask a sufferer of RLS whether it is a real disease or born out of vivid imagination. The suffering and agony of many a severely afflicted RLS patient will tell the true story. Numerous scientific papers published in peer-reviewed journals and chapters in textbooks dealing with RLS in the last 20 years or so attest to the fact that RLS is a real neurological movement disorder severely impacting sleep and quality of life. Unfortunately, we do not yet have a laboratory test to confirm the diagnosis, nor do we know the exact cause of the condition. We are making progress in both directions. In the meantime, fortunately, effective drug treatment is available to relieve the suffering of many unfortunate victims. The RLS community (both the professionals and lay organizations including the RLS Foundation) has been trying to educate the public and the profession about the nature of RLS, and it is making progress slowly but steadily. National Institutes of Health (NIH) through the National Center for Sleep Disorders Research (NCSDR) have been encouraging and supporting research in RLS and this is good news.

In this book, directed at patients (and which may also prove useful for family physicians and other non-RLS specialists), I have tried to discuss the nature of the condition, its clinical presentation, the diagnostic criteria, management, and the forthcoming developments in new treatment. The success of this endeavor will depend on how you, the readers, view this contribution.

I must acknowledge several individuals who made the publication of this book possible. First I thank Christopher Davis, Executive Publisher of Medicine at Jones & Bartlett Learning, for his professionalism and helpful attitude. Leah Corrigan, Associate Production Editor, and others at Jones & Bartlett Learning also deserve my thanks for their help in publishing, copyediting, and marketing this book. I thank Annabella Drennan, the Editorial Assistant to *Sleep Medicine* journal, for editing and making corrections; Betty Coram for typing the initial draft of the entire book; and Jenny Rodriguez for typing some parts of the book. I also give special thanks to Mark Mahowald, MD, and Cynthia Comella, MD, for making thoughtful comments about the book. Last but not least, I must thank my wife, Manisha Chokroverty, MD, not only for her continued support, patience, and love during every stage of production of the book, but also for her insight into the condition and for suggesting some of the questions. I am indebted to all my patients from whom I have learned a great deal about RLS and who vividly described many aspects of the condition which cannot be learned by reading the books and journals.

PART ONE

The Basics

What is restless legs syndrome?

How common is RLS?

What causes RLS?

More . . .

1. What is restless legs syndrome?

Restless legs syndrome (RLS) is a sensorimotor neurologic and movement disorder that seriously impacts sleep and quality of life. The patient experiences characteristic complaints of unpleasant sensations in the legs with an urge to move while lying down in bed at night trying to get to sleep; these sensations are relieved by movement, at least temporarily. RLS is thought to be the most common neurological movement disorder most uncommonly diagnosed. Indeed, this condition is often misdiagnosed and misunderstood. Many times in the past, patients with RLS were labeled as "psychoneurotics." More recently, there has been significant awareness of the condition in contemporary medicine, although some people continue to mislabel RLS as a "disease-mongering" condition. These skeptics really should take the time to ask persons with RLS (those suffering from moderately severe to severe disease) what the condition is like. To these individuals, RLS is a torture. Some have even stated, "I would rather die than live with this dreaded disease." Recent studies have clearly shown that RLS is a real disease with a biological basis and that it is familial, is associated with many other disorders, and can be treated effectively if diagnosed correctly and differentiated from other conditions mimicking RLS.

The name "restless legs syndrome" itself does not evoke the true seriousness of this condition. Often the disease is not taken seriously because the patient does not necessarily look sick and generally remains symptom free in the daytime. One of the problems in defining RLS is that there is no single laboratory test that can definitively prove the presence of the disease; instead, the diagnosis depends entirely on patients' symptoms and physicians' critical evaluation of these

Restless legs syndrome (RLS)

A sensorimotor neurologic and movement disorder that seriously affects sleep and quality of life.

symptoms. Many patients do not seek advice of the physicians because they are apprehensive that their symptoms will not be taken seriously and that they will be labeled as psychoneurotics.

RLS is a very common disease (see Question 2) that may affect as much as 10% of the population; the most severe disease requiring physician intervention may affect 2.7% of the population. RLS is associated with significant **morbidity** (illness of health) that affects the person's quality of life, interferes with social and personal relationships, and makes day-to-day functioning difficult (and the affected person miserable). Sleep dysfunction is a major complaint of affected patients; this problem may coexist with anxiety, depression, obesity, heart failure, excessive daytime sleepiness, and impairment of cognition, concentration, affect, and attention.

Morbidity
Illness of health.

2. How common is RLS?

RLS is a very common disorder. Unfortunately, because of misconceptions and lack of adequate knowledge about RLS, this condition remains underdiagnosed or goes undiagnosed. The diagnosis is based on the essential criteria outlined in Question 4, which are based on the patient's history and physical examination. Before the essential criteria for diagnosis were defined, any patients with restlessness were often diagnosed as having RLS or suffering from a psychoneurotic disorder. For this reason, the number of cases diagnosed before the essential criteria were agreed upon is considered unreliable.

Unfortunately, because of misconceptions and lack of adequate knowledge about RLS, this condition remains underdiagnosed or goes undiagnosed.

Surveys from North American, Northern European, and Western European populations, taking into consideration the essential criteria (see Question 4), have shown the **prevalence** as varying from 2.5% to 10%.

Prevalence
The number of cases of a disease, whether old or new, existing within a given population at a stated point in time.

The Basics

The prevalence of more severe cases (people who have symptoms at least twice weekly with distress) is approximately 2.7%. Some surveys have found a lower prevalence, suggesting a possible ethnic and racial difference in RLS prevalence. In surveys from some Asian countries (e.g., South Korea), the prevalence found was similar to that observed in Western countries.

The differences in the prevalence rates may be due to factors other than ethnic and racial differences. For example, local environmental factors (e.g., a particular diet, presence of toxins in the environment, lifestyle factors) may play a role in the development of RLS. These issues have not been definitively identified, however, and have not been addressed adequately in different surveys. Some of the known risk factors associated with RLS are increasing age, female gender, pregnancy, iron deficiency, **neuropathy** (damage to peripheral nerves), and end-stage kidney disease (see **Table 1**).

Neuropathy
Damage to peripheral nerves.

Table 1 Risk Factors for Restless Legs Syndrome

Population Characteristics
• Increasing age
• Female gender
• Lower socioeconomic status
• Residents of North America and Western and Northern Europe

Physiological Factors
• Pregnancy
• Poor physical and general health

Lifestyle Factors (Preventable)
• Smoking
• Inactive lifestyle
• Obesity from overeating
• High-altitude living
• Alcohol use

Medical and Neurological Disorders (See Question 40)

Family History of RLS

Up until recently, all of the studies of RLS have addressed prevalence (i.e., the number of cases, whether old or new, existing within a given population at a stated point in time). No study is available to ascertain **incidence** (i.e., the number of new cases in a given population during a stated period). Furthermore, all of the investigations involving RLS have addressed the severity of the disease based on standardized scales (see Question 32), but have not adequately addressed the severity based on frequency and intensity of symptoms. For example, a patient with frequent (occurring three to four times per week in the evening or daytime), severe symptoms is certainly different from a patient with an occasional symptom (occurring once every few weeks) of short duration. Various surveys have shown that 20% of the patients will have daily or almost daily symptoms, 40% will have symptoms at least weekly (one to three times per week) but not daily, and 40% will have symptoms every few weeks or months (less than weekly symptoms).

Incidence

The number of new cases in a given population during a stated period.

The Basics

3. Is RLS a disease of the contemporary time or was it known in earlier times?

The term "restless legs syndrome" was coined by Karl Ekbom, a Swedish physician, in 1944. Ekbom later gave a masterful description of the condition in a monograph in 1945. He not only described the uncomfortable feelings in the legs and motor restlessness associated with movements during sleep, but also mentioned the positive family history of RLS, association with pregnancy, iron deficiency, anemia, gastric surgery, and malabsorption of vitamin B_{12} as well as patients' positive responses to treatment with opium. Thus, RLS is not a new disease of contemporary medicine, though it has been recently rediscovered and we are now more enlightened about this condition.

Most sleep scientists believe that the first description of the illness now called RLS was probably given by the great English physician Thomas Willis, who first described this condition in Latin in 1672; his work was translated into English in 1683. Willis described the condition as follows:

Wherefore to some, when being a bed, betake themselves to sleep presently in the arms and legs, leapings and contractions of the tendons, and so great a restlessness and tossing of their members ensue, that the diseased are no more able to sleep, than if they were in a place of greatest torture.

This description seems similar to the descriptions of RLS patients found in the contemporary literature. A search through the literature, including philosophical and religious writings, however, indicates that RLS was known to the Greeks and even centuries earlier in the Vedic literature of the Hindu religion. Nevertheless, the description by Ekbom in the middle of the last century was the catalyst that brought this condition to the forefront of the medical community.

Unfortunately, the scientific community had to wait nearly two centuries after the description by Willis before Wittmack described RLS-like symptoms under the heading of "anxietias tibiarum" (anxiety state) in 1861. Both Beard in 1918 and Oppenheim in 1923 used the term "neurasthenia" (weakness of nerves) to describe what appeared to be RLS-like symptoms. The descriptions of leg movements caused by paresthesia (a skin sensation such as burning or tingling) during rest by Mussio-Fournier and Rawak in 1940 and of "leg jitters" by Allison in 1943 preceded the introduction of the notion of "irritable legs" by Ekbom in 1944 and finally the term "restless legs" in 1945.

The next milestone in the history of RLS came from a group led by Lugaresi in Bologna, Italy, in 1965. These researchers made physiological recordings of periodic leg movements in sleep (see Question 34) found in at least 80% of patients with RLS. Nearly 20 years later, a major advance in treatment of RLS came from the serendipitous observation of Akpinar, a Turkish physician; in 1982, he observed improvement of RLS in a patient with **Parkinson's disease** (a degenerative disorder of the central nervous system that often impairs the sufferer's motor skills, speech, and posture) after treatment with levodopa.

The establishment of the RLS Foundation in 1992 and the International RLS Study Group (IRLSSG) in 1995 acted as a catalyst for education and awareness of RLS in contemporary medicine. Increasing awareness of this very common condition eventually attracted the attention of the pharmaceutical companies and prompted them to begin developing drugs for RLS, including conducting clinical trials with these medications. Following these trials, in both North America and Europe, two drugs were officially approved for treatment of RLS: ropinirole in 2005 and pramipexole in 2007. Active research into RLS continues throughout the world to understand what causes RLS. Although we are making slow but continuous progress, as yet we have not found the cause of the disease.

4. How do physicians diagnose RLS?

Currently, there is no single laboratory diagnostic test available for RLS. Therefore, the diagnosis is based entirely on an analysis of the patient's symptoms. A few years ago, a group of physicians from North America, Europe, and other parts of the world who had a special interest in RLS (including the author of this book)

The Basics

Parkinson's disease

A degenerative disorder of the central nervous system that often impairs the sufferer's motor skills, speech, and posture.

Active research into RLS continues throughout the world to understand what causes RLS.

began an effort to develop some minimal clinical criteria for making a diagnosis of RLS. Development of such criteria, it was thought, would enable scientists to design good epidemiological studies for RLS and would standardize the definition of RLS for research purposes. In 1995, the International Restless Legs Syndrome Study Group (IRLSSG) published four essential criteria for the diagnosis of RLS; these criteria were slightly modified in a later National Institutes of Health Consensus Conference and were published in 2003 in *Sleep Medicine*, an international sleep medical journal. These essential criteria are summarized in **Table 2** and explained at length here. All four of the essential criteria must be met with or without the supportive and associated features (described below).

Criterion 1: Individuals suffering from RLS develop an intense, disagreeable feeling, variously described as creeping, crawling, tingling, burning, painful, aching, cramping, vise-like, or itchy, much like bugs crawling under the skin or water running under the skin. The uncomfortable sensations occur mostly between the

Table 2   Four Essential Criteria for the Diagnosis of RLS

- **Criterion 1:** an urge to move the legs, usually accompanied or caused by unpleasant or uncomfortable, sometimes indescribable sensations in the legs. Sometimes the urge to move is present without these uncomfortable sensations and, in some patients, the arms or other body parts are involved in addition to the legs.
- **Criterion 2:** the urge to move or unpleasant sensations begin or worsen during periods of rest or inactivity such as lying down or sitting.
- **Criterion 3:** the urge to move or unpleasant sensations are partially or totally relieved by movements such as walking or stretching, at least as long as the activity continues.
- **Criterion 4:** the urge to move or unpleasant sensations are worse in the evening or at night than during the day or occur exclusively in the evening or at night. In case of long-standing and severe RLS, the worsening of symptoms at night may not be noticeable but must have been present previously.

knees and ankles, causing an intense urge to move the legs to relieve these feelings. In some patients, the pain begins in the thighs or the feet. Sometimes patients complain of similar symptoms in the arms or other body parts (the hips, trunk, shoulders, genitals, anal regions, and, extremely rarely, the face). The symptoms in the legs usually occur first and then the patient may complain of symptoms in other body parts later. Symptoms generally occur in both legs, but sometimes may occur in one leg or the symptoms may alternate between the two legs. About 20% to 25% of patients with RLS complain of actual pain. In some patients, especially in the early stages of the disease, the symptoms may occur occasionally, perhaps once a week. Later, as the disease progresses, symptoms may occur two to three times per week or even daily, and the intensity of the symptoms may also increase later in the course of the illness.

Criterion 2: Rest provokes symptom onset. RLS is a disease of **quiescence**. That is, when a patient is tired and trying to get to sleep, the symptoms begin and peak. At least in the beginning stages of the disease, the symptoms do not occur immediately on rest, but rather appear a few minutes after lying down or resting. As the disease progresses or if the patient develops what is called **augmentation** (see Questions 73 and 74), the latency between resting and the onset of symptom decreases or, in severe cases, symptoms appear immediately on lying down and the symptom intensity increases.

Criterion 3: Getting up from bed can immediately relieve the symptoms (at least partially) as long as the patient is up and moving and walking. Many patients try all types of tricks to obtain relief from the condition.

The Basics

Quiescence
Being still or inactive; being at rest.

Augmentation
Drug-induced complications first noted with levodopa treatment, consisting of earlier onset of symptoms and intensification of symptoms that spread to other body parts.

They move, massage, or rub their legs; they get out of bed to walk around. These maneuvers may temporarily relieve the symptoms. For some individuals, warm baths may prove helpful. In the most severe cases, symptoms may even occur in the daytime when patients are sitting or lying down. Long travel by car, train, or plane may be particularly distressing. Many individuals with RLS find it impossible to sit for any length of time in a movie house or theater. They find that they must stand in the back of the theater to relieve the intense disagreeable feelings in their legs. Patients also find that distraction or intense mental activity (playing games, watching an exciting movie, engaging in a heated discussion) provides relief from the intense disagreeable feelings and the urge to move the legs.

Criterion 4: Most patients find that their symptoms are worse in the evening or during the night, or occur exclusively during these periods. In advanced cases with more progression of the disease, symptoms may occur toward the end of the day; symptoms may also be severe without any preferences for the evening period. It is now conclusively established that RLS symptoms follow a true **circadian** (*circa* means "about," *dian* means "day") pattern, with the most severe symptoms occurring between 10 P.M. and 4 A.M. and often marked relief being noted between 7 A.M. and 11 A.M. This pattern persists even in individuals whose work schedule may include an unconventional sleep–wake cycle (e.g., shift workers).

Circadian

Occurring in a roughly 24-hour cycle.

The IRLSSG consensus conference also identified some supportive and associated features of RLS (**Table 3**) to help make a diagnosis in those cases where patients are not able to clearly describe their symptoms and because the physicians are not always certain whether symptoms

Table 3   Supportive and Associated Features of RLS

Supportive Clinical Features
- Response to dopaminergic medications (see Question 71)
- Familial occurrence of RLS (see Question 7)
- Abnormal movements of the legs causing periodic limb movements in sleep (PLMS) as well as periodic limb movements in wakefulness (PLMW) (see Question 34)

Associated Features of RLS
- Sleep disturbances (see Question 27)
- Normal neurological examination in those cases of RLS where it is not associated with other conditions and no causes are found
- Usually a chronic progressive course (see Question 16)

fulfill all four of the essential criteria (see Table 2). With patients who do not fulfill all the essential criteria because of uncertainty about the symptoms or confusion of RLS symptoms with other conditions resembling RLS, the supportive clinical features listed in Table 3 may help in establishing a diagnosis.

As noted in Table 3, almost all patients with RLS respond to a dopaminergic medication, which is generally given in much smaller doses for RLS than for Parkinson's disease. This response is initially positive but may not be universally maintained later on. For documenting periodic limb movements in sleep (PLMS) or periodic limb movements in wakefulness (PLMW) (see Question 34), an overnight physiological recording (polysomnographic recording; see Question 31) is needed. PLMS is present in at least 80% of RLS patients but not in 100%; thus it is not considered a specific diagnostic test for RLS. Approximately 60% of patients with RLS have a positive family history of RLS (see Question 7).

In a recent study performed at Johns Hopkins University, researchers demonstrated that up to 16% of individuals

The Basics

False positive

A result that appears to be positive (indicating the presence of disease) when it is actually normal (no disease).

Central nervous system (CNS)

The brain and the spinal cord.

Cerebral hemisphere

The main part of the brain. The right cerebral hemisphere controls the left side of the body; the left cerebral hemisphere controls the right side of the body.

Brain stem

The lower part of the brain, which is connected to the main portion of the brain and controls vital functions such as circulation, respiration, and sleep.

Spinal cord

The long tubular structure of the central nervous system that connects to the brain stem and runs through the vertebral column.

without RLS may satisfy all the four diagnostic criteria for RLS, giving rise to **false positive** cases. The RLS specialists, therefore, started a conversation about the possibility of adding another criterion to discriminate RLS from those conditions that closely mimic RLS. Consensus has not yet been reached about which features differentiate these so-called mimetics from true RLS (see Question 39 for more on these conditions).

5. What causes RLS?

Researchers have been trying to find the cause of RLS since Ekbom's description of this condition appeared 65 years ago. Today we know a great deal about RLS—but not exactly what causes RLS or which part of the nervous system, if any, is affected. It is generally thought that RLS is a disorder arising from the **central nervous system (CNS)**, even though no specific structural abnormality has been identified. Is the problem located in the **cerebral hemisphere** (the main part of the brain), the **brain stem** (the lower part of the brain, which is connected to the main portion of the brain and controls vital functions such as circulation, respiration, and sleep), or the **spinal cord** (the long tubular structure of the CNS that connects to the brain stem and runs through the vertebral column)? Various studies indicate probable involvement of all levels of the CNS. No structural alteration in the cells or the connections of the CNS has so far been noted. Thus, RLS most likely results from a functional—rather than a structural—abnormality in some site of the CNS.

Based on research studies, it appears that the problem lies somewhere between the main portion of the brain and the spinal cord. Patients' response to RLS treatments and other studies point to a problem with a chemical called **dopamine**, a neurotransmitter made in the nerve cells that helps transmit nerve impulses to other nerve cells. Dopamine is deficient in Parkinson's disease—there is loss of cells manufacturing dopamine in Parkinson's disease. The problem with dopamine in patients with RLS, however, seems to involve a different mechanism than is present in Parkinson's disease. The results do not clearly show that dopamine is deficient in RLS. Perhaps there is a wide variation of dopamine levels between day and night, with a marked decline in levels occurring in the evening and during the night in RLS patients.

The contemporary thinking or understanding of RLS suggests that this disease may be caused by an abnormality in the body's use and storage of iron, at least in a subgroup of RLS patients. Iron is needed for dopamine synthesis; consequently, a deficiency of iron in the brain may contribute to the dopamine dysfunction. Iron deficiency aggravates RLS symptoms, and iron treatment in these patients ameliorates these symptoms, suggesting a role for iron in RLS. Low stores of iron in the brain and dysfunction of iron metabolism and intracellular iron may play key roles in RLS pathophysiology. This iron–dopamine model suggests that brain iron deficiency causes an abnormality in the dopaminergic system, in turn leading to RLS symptoms.

Neurophysiological and functional magnetic resonance imaging (fMRI) studies suggest that the dysfunction may occur somewhere in the region of the brain stem. In most cases of RLS, however, no clear cause is found.

In some patients, RLS symptoms may arise secondary to other disorders, such as an abnormality of the nerves

Dopamine

A neurotransmitter made in the nerve cells that helps transmit nerve impulses to other nerve cells.

The Basics

Kidneys

The pair of organs that is responsible for urine production and excretion from the body.

Because we do not know the exact cause of RLS, we can only treat the symptoms but not cure the disease at present.

conducting impulses outside the CNS, chronic failure of the **kidneys** (the organs responsible for urine production and excretion from the body), iron deficiency, diabetes mellitus, or chronic joint disease (see Question 14). RLS may also be associated with or caused by some medications (e.g., antidepressants, antihistamines; see Question 82). Because we do not know the exact cause of RLS, we can only treat the symptoms but not cure the disease at present. The good news is that most patients get relief, although they may have to continue taking medication indefinitely.

PART TWO

Risk, Prevention, and Epidemiology of Restless Legs Syndrome

My mother has RLS. I am a 35-year-old woman. Could I get RLS from my mother?

If I am diagnosed with RLS during pregnancy, what are my chances of having this condition permanently?

Does a patient with RLS develop Parkinson's disease later in life?

More . . .

6. I am a 65-year-old woman. For the past two years, I have been having restless feelings in my legs when lying down in bed at night. My friend says I may have RLS. Is my friend correct?

It is appropriate to consider RLS when any person complains of restless feelings in the legs while lying down in bed at night. The diagnosis of RLS, as discussed in Question 4, depends entirely on the patient's symptoms. The characteristic feature is an urge to move the legs, most often as a result of disagreeable, uncomfortable feelings in the legs (occasionally, patients may not have these disagreeable feelings in the legs) when resting in bed or while relaxing in the evening. If you have these symptoms only or predominantly in the evening, and moving the legs, rubbing the legs, or getting out of bed and walking around the bed relieves the symptoms at least temporarily, then your symptoms are highly suggestive of RLS. The symptoms may come as soon as you lie down in bed, so that you may have to get out of bed again and exercise the legs before coming back to bed. This may happen several times, disturbing your sleep and making it difficult for you to fall asleep. As a result you may have difficulty functioning in the daytime because of sleep deprivation.

Often, there is a comorbid condition or cause associated with the development of RLS.

In older patients, symptoms of RLS tend to be fairly rapidly progressive and may become worse within the next five years. Often, there is a comorbid condition or cause associated with the development of RLS (see Question 40). You should definitely consult a physician specializing in sleep medicine and particularly RLS for confirming the diagnosis. Effective treatment is available so that patients do not have to suffer from these uncomfortable feelings and having to move the legs at bedtime, disturbing their sleep for days, weeks, or months.

7. My mother has RLS. I am a 35-year-old woman. Could I get RLS from my mother?

Several family studies of RLS suggest an increased occurrence (as much as 60%) in first-degree relatives of **idiopathic** RLS cases (those not associated with other diseases and for which no causes are found). The presence of similar symptoms in such a high percentage of patients suggests that RLS follows a dominant mode of inheritance. As a consequence, half the siblings are at increased risk for developing RLS. First- and second-degree relatives of RLS patients are affected more often than controls. It is estimated that the first-degree relatives of RLS patients are five times more likely to have RLS than the nonrelatives. This risk is particularly apparent in patients with an early age of onset of RLS (before the age of 45 years).

Idiopathic case

A case not associated with other diseases and for which no cause is found.

Many studies do indicate that RLS runs in families, although this finding may be due to either familial occurrence or a shared common environmental factor. As yet, researchers have not precisely determined the exact risk of RLS occurring in close relatives. The recent genome-wide association study for RLS identified common variants in certain genomic regions, confirming more than a 50% increase in risk for RLS in persons with these variants. Various investigators have examined the DNA in chromosomes and discovered a similar genetic makeup in people with RLS, and one that is different from the genetic makeup of those persons who do not have RLS. These studies have pointed to several locations in the chromosomes that might hold genes responsible for RLS, although no specific genes have been uncovered as yet.

It is clear from the various studies that RLS is a complex disorder that may result from a number of genetic and environmental factors. Therefore, it is not possible to give an absolute answer as to whether you will inherit RLS from your mother, but you do have a greater chance of doing so than persons whose parents do not have RLS.

8. I am a 50-year-old man with diabetic neuropathy (nerve damage). Sometimes I get uncomfortable feelings in my legs and an urge to move while I'm resting. Are these symptoms due to nerve damage as a result of diabetes or do I have another condition?

The question here is whether you have symptoms due to diabetic neuropathy or whether you have symptoms that may suggest another condition such as RLS. In cases of long-term **diabetes mellitus**, damage to the peripheral nerves may cause symptoms of tingling, numbness, burning, and stabbing, generally in a "stocking and glove" distribution. These sensory symptoms are present intermittently or throughout the day, but do not necessarily become worse in the evenings; also, they are generally *not* relieved by movements. In addition, patients with diabetes mellitus may experience weakness of the muscles of the legs, which does not occur in RLS. RLS is thought to be more common in persons with diabetes mellitus than in the general population. Indeed, several case series have recently shown that RLS occurs more frequently in diabetes patients, particularly in those who develop diabetic neuropathy.

The sensory symptoms of patients with primary RLS are characterized by deep, disagreeable, unpleasant,

Diabetes mellitus

A condition in which a person has a high glucose (blood sugar) level, either because the body fails to produce enough insulin or because the cells do not properly respond to the insulin that is produced.

often nonlocalized and nonradiating discomfort accompanied by no objective sensory impairment. In contrast, diabetic peripheral neuropathy patients often show impairment of sensation on objective testing. It is also notable that in about 20 to 25% of patients with primary RLS, there is actual pain rather than intense disagreeable feelings. The difficulty in distinguishing between the two situations arises in those patients who are genetically predisposed to develop RLS symptoms: In such a case, the patient may have mixed diabetic neuropathic and RLS sensory symptoms.

As mentioned in Question 4, RLS patients' complaints should meet all four essential diagnostic criteria. Therefore, it is possible to have both diabetic peripheral neuropathy and RLS. To make the diagnosis in this case, the patient should consult a neurologist who is also a sleep specialist, particularly a neurologist with special interest in RLS.

9. I am 7 months pregnant. Recently I noticed that I get strange feelings in my legs with an urge to move my legs in the evening while resting in bed. A friend who has RLS tells me that I may be developing symptoms of RLS. Is my friend correct?

Your friend may very well be correct. You should consult an RLS specialist as well as your obstetrician/gynecologist. Several studies have found an increased frequency of RLS during pregnancy. Approximately 20 to 25% of expectant mothers develop RLS during pregnancy, most prominently in the last trimester of pregnancy. Interestingly, Ekbom (who originally coined the term "restless legs syndrome" and described this

Approximately 20 to 25% of expectant mothers develop RLS during pregnancy, most prominently in the last trimester of pregnancy.

disease's clinical features in the middle of the twentieth century) reported a high prevalence of RLS symptoms in pregnant women. In some pregnant women with a previous diagnosis of RLS, symptoms become worse during pregnancy; in the majority, however, symptoms appear for the first time during pregnancy with subsequent resolution of symptoms around the time of delivery. Some studies have noted worsening of previously experienced RLS symptoms or the onset of RLS symptoms for the first time during pregnancy in both familial and nonfamilial RLS patients, albeit more frequently in cases of familial RLS. Several factors are thought to be responsible for the exacerbation or occurrence of RLS symptoms during pregnancy, including iron and folate deficiencies (although folic acid or folate is now prescribed routinely throughout pregnancy), hormonal changes (e.g., increased levels of estrogen, progesterone, and prolactin), and mechanical factors causing lower limb vascular congestion.

10. If I am diagnosed with RLS during pregnancy, what are my chances of having this condition permanently?

In most pregnant women with newly developed RLS, symptoms will resolve near the time of delivery. In a small minority, symptoms will persist after delivery, suggesting that the pregnancy might have triggered RLS in those who are genetically predisposed to develop this condition. In those patients who have previously diagnosed RLS, symptoms may become worse during pregnancy but will improve after delivery; such patients may continue to have symptoms with the same frequency and intensity as noted prior to becoming pregnant.

11. I have chronic kidney problems. I have started experiencing symptoms of restlessness in the legs in the evening while I am lying in bed trying to get to sleep. Am I developing symptoms of RLS? How common is RLS in kidney failure?

Studies have generally found an increased frequency of RLS (20 to 50% or even higher) in patients with severe kidney failure or end-stage kidney disease, particularly those on dialysis (15 to 70%). There is an ethnic variation in this pattern: Patients from Northern Europe with severe kidney failure have a higher prevalence than similar patients from India and Japan. The clinical features of RLS in patients with kidney failure are similar to those noted in patients with idiopathic RLS. Some studies, however, suggest that patients with severe kidney failure may have more severe RLS symptoms and more severe sleep disturbances than those with mild kidney failure. There is also a suggestion of increased frequency of deaths in those kidney failure patients who have RLS as compared to those who do not have RLS.

No specific factors have been identified to explain the high frequency of RLS in patients with kidney failure, although it has been suggested that anemia, iron deficiency, and peripheral nerve damage as a result of kidney failure may play roles. It has not been determined whether aggressive treatment of iron deficiency in patients with severe kidney failure will decrease the severity of their symptoms as well as their morbidity and mortality. A sleep specialist with experience in RLS will be the best physician to answer questions about whether a person with kidney disease is developing RLS symptoms.

12. I am a 60-year-old man with Parkinson's disease on levodopa treatment. Recently, I noticed an urge to move my legs while I am in bed trying to get to sleep. Am I developing RLS symptoms? How common is RLS in patients with Parkinson's disease?

The relationship between RLS and Parkinson's disease (PD) remains somewhat controversial. Both RLS and PD patients benefit from dopaminergic medications, although RLS patients need much lower doses of these medications compared to PD patients. In many respects, however, these two conditions are quite different.

Some brain neuroimaging studies show a very mild dysfunction of the **basal ganglia** (groups of nerve cells and connecting fibers and neurons located deep in the brain that control movements, gait, posture, and emotions); however, other studies have failed to find any such abnormalities. In contrast, in PD patients, there is severe dysfunction of these structures with marked loss of neurons. In RLS patients, no such loss of neurons has been described. RLS patients show evidence of decreased iron storage in these structures, whereas PD patients exhibit increased iron accumulation.

Earlier studies showed no increased prevalence of RLS in PD. Some recent studies, however, have identified an increased prevalence of RLS in PD patients. It has been noted that most RLS symptoms in PD patients begin after treatment with dopaminergic medications, indicating that perhaps RLS may develop in these PD patients through a mechanism of augmentation (see Question 74). There may be an increased prevalence of RLS in PD patients, but without further studies, it is not possible to draw any definitive conclusions at this

Basal ganglia

Groups of nerve cells and connecting fibers and neurons located deep in the brain that control movements, gait, posture, and emotions.

stage. Your sleep doctor should be able to tell you whether you are developing symptoms of RLS, based on the essential RLS diagnostic criteria (see Question 4).

13. Does a patient with RLS develop Parkinson's disease later in life?

At the present time, there is no evidence that a patient with RLS will develop PD later in life. Keep in mind, however, that PD and RLS are both fairly common disorders in later life, and sometimes the two conditions may exist together by chance. To answer this question definitively, what is needed is a good epidemiologic study comparing a large number of age- and sex-matched control subjects and RLS and PD patients to show the prevalence of PD in RLS and determine how many RLS patients will later develop PD.

At the present time, there is no evidence that a patient with RLS will develop PD later in life.

14. I suffer from rheumatoid arthritis. I experience pain and indescribable uncomfortable feelings in my legs in the evening while resting. A friend told me that I may have RLS. Is this true? How common is RLS in patients with rheumatoid arthritis?

Two early reports in the 1990s directed our attention to the possibility of increasing prevalence of RLS in patients with rheumatoid arthritis. There has been a resurgence of this hypothesis in recent literature, although contradictory reports on this possibility also exist. Overall, it is believed that there is an increasing prevalence of RLS in rheumatologic disorders including rheumatoid arthritis. Nevertheless, it is important to differentiate RLS symptoms from the pain and discomfort associated with arthritis, as some of the symptoms of these two conditions may be similar. In patients with arthritis, the pain and discomfort are limited to the joints; this pain may become more intense in the evening, mimicking RLS. The pain and discomfort in RLS improve on walking. In contrast, in arthritis, the pain becomes worse when walking. Furthermore, the uncomfortable feelings in RLS are limited not just to the joints but occur most commonly in the legs between the knees and ankles, although other body parts may be involved. Physicians taking care of patients suffering from rheumatologic disorders should be aware of the four essential diagnostic criteria for RLS (see Question 4) so that they can effectively differentiate between RLS and arthritic conditions.

15. I am a 59-year-old man who has been experiencing restlessness of the whole body throughout the day. I cannot sit still; I keep moving all the time. I have been taking a neuroleptic medication for a "nervous breakdown." My friend looked up my symptoms on the Internet and told me that I have RLS. Is this true?

RLS certainly needs to be considered in this scenario, although RLS symptoms—at least in the beginning—are not present throughout the day. RLS symptoms initially occur in the evening or are present exclusively in the evening; as the disease progresses into advanced stages, however, patients may have symptoms in the daytime.

Akathisia

A "subjective desire to be in constant motion" associated with "an inability to sit or stand still" and a "drive to pace up and down" [FDA definition].

In this case, the symptoms point to another condition that is often mistaken for RLS and that commonly occurs as a long-term side effect of neuroleptic medications—namely, **akathisia** (derived from the Greek word meaning "inability to sit"). There are two essential features of akathisia: a subjective feeling of inner restlessness and an objective feature of motor restlessness, which is most commonly induced by **neuroleptic** (nerve-calming) medications. A U.S. Food and Drug Administration (FDA) Task Force defined akathisia as a "subjective desire to be in constant motion" associated with "an inability to sit or stand still" and a "drive to pace up and down." The inner feeling of restlessness or fidgetiness causes forced walking. As a result, a person with akathisia may have difficulty sitting still and may keep moving, crossing and uncrossing the legs, swaying and rocking back and forth, and constantly shifting body positions during sitting.

Neuroleptic
Nerve-calming medication.

In akathisia, the whole body is in restless motion; in RLS, the urge to move while restless is limited to the legs. Another feature that differentiates akathisia from RLS is that the movements of restlessness in akathisia are present throughout the day but may become worse in the evening. There is no *pattern* of worsening or exclusive presentation of the symptoms in the evening, however—unlike that noted in RLS. Finally, the movements in akathisia do not occur as a result of an urge to move preceded by discomfort, unlike that noted in RLS. The fundamental feature of RLS is presence or worsening of symptoms during inactivity or quiescence. In contrast, in akathisia, the movements are present not only during inactivity, but also while standing and walking, as if the whole body is in constant motion. Patients with akathisia also do not complain of uncomfortable or disagreeable sensations in the legs (except in rare cases).

The most important feature in this scenario is that the patient has been taking a neuroleptic medication, which is most likely causing the symptoms of restlessness rather than RLS. Therefore, it is unlikely that this patient has RLS. Note, however, that in advanced stages of RLS, some patients may complain of generalized restlessness involving the whole body without obtaining any significant relief from the movements, making it difficult to differentiate this type of RLS from akathisia. Such patients will have a prior history of characteristic symptoms fulfilling all the four essential criteria for RLS (see Question 4).

16. I have RLS that is moderately controlled on medication (see Question 71). Will I have RLS all my life or does the medication cure the disease?

This very important question focuses on the course and natural history of RLS. RLS is generally considered a chronic disorder with a progressive course. Although some patients will experience intermittent remissions of symptoms for weeks to months, overall the disease progresses over time. The course of the disease is usually more slowly progressive in those who develop symptoms at an earlier age (younger than 45 years) than in those persons whose symptoms first appear at a later age. The patients presenting to the physicians at a later age generally experience a more rapid course, and the RLS is often associated with **comorbid** conditions that may have been responsible for or aggravated the RLS.

Comorbid
Coexisting.

In the family history study conducted at Johns Hopkins University Hospital, more than 95% of those patients interviewed had the disease for an average of almost 20 years. It is important for the physicians caring for RLS to remember the chronicity of the condition and to appreciate that RLS is similar to some other chronic medical conditions, such as hypertension and diabetes mellitus, requiring monitoring and treatment throughout the patient's entire life.

17. My 8-year-old child was diagnosed with "growing pains." Is this a correct diagnosis or can he have RLS?

The diagnosis of growing pains in a child may be a problematic one, as some patients with the diagnosis of growing pains may actually be experiencing RLS symptoms. A subgroup of patients have been diagnosed as having both conditions simultaneously. There is also a general misperception that RLS is an adult disease and does not occur in children. Thus, even if the child does have characteristic symptoms of RLS fulfilling all four of the essential criteria (see Question 4), the condition may mistakenly be diagnosed as "growing pains." Some of these patients may also be mistakenly diagnosed with attention-deficit/hyperactivity disorder (ADHD) because of fidgetiness (see Question 18).

There is also a general misperception that RLS is an adult disease and does not occur in children.

Growing pains generally occur in early and late childhood and are characterized by pain that is often stabbing; this pain typically occurs before the child falls asleep or when he or she is waking up from sleep. It predominantly affects the thigh and the calf muscles. As in RLS, these patients may obtain pain relief from massage or cold or warm baths. Growing pain symptoms are not relieved by movements. Parents should consult a pediatric neurologist or a sleep specialist to clarify whether their child truly has growing pains or is developing RLS symptoms.

18. My 6-year-old child is always fidgety and restless. Does he have attention-deficit/hyperactivity disorder or can he have RLS?

Attention-deficit/hyperactivity disorder (ADHD) is characterized by fidgetiness and excessive motor restlessness, in addition to inattention and, in some patients,

Attention-deficit/ hyperactivity disorder (ADHD)

A disorder characterized by fidgetiness, excessive motor restlessness, inattention, and (in some patients) impulsivity.

impulsivity. Any restlessness in a child is not necessarily ADHD; in fact, this condition is often diagnosed in error. Sometimes it is mistaken for RLS, or the true RLS symptoms are mistaken for ADHD.

The Diagnostic and Statistical Manual of Mental Disorders, revised fourth edition (*DSM-IV-TR*), published in 2000 by the American Psychiatric Association, listed diagnostic criteria for ADHD. These criteria include six or more symptoms of inattention or hyperactivity and/or impulsivity for at least six months, with the symptoms not being consistent with the developmental level of the child. The symptoms are present before age seven years, and affected children show impairment in two or more settings (e.g., at home or at school). There is clear evidence of interference with the development of appropriate social, academic, or occupational functioning, and the disturbance is not explained by another mental disorder.

Restlessness, inattention, and hyperactivity in some RLS patients may resemble ADHD, and these symptoms may have been caused by chronic sleep deprivation in RLS. Therefore, whether these symptoms suggest an association between RLS and ADHD or are simply the result of chronic sleep disturbance remains to be determined.

19. How do physicians diagnose RLS in children who may not be able to describe their symptoms adequately?

Children may not be able to describe RLS symptoms accurately. As a consequence, they are often misdiagnosed as having growing pains or ADHD. Children will describe the symptoms in their own language (e.g., childish language such as "ouch," "owies," or "boo-boos");

their inability to give an accurate description initially led researchers to believe that RLS did not occur in children. Upon questioning, however, many adult RLS patients describe their symptoms as beginning in childhood and progressing very slowly over the years.

To address this problem, a National Institutes of Health (NIH) Workshop in 2002 established diagnostic criteria specifically for children between an arbitrary age limit of 2 to 12 years (see **Table 4**); these criteria were published in *Sleep Medicine*, an international journal dealing with clinical sleep disorders, in 2003. The criteria for children include all of the adult essential diagnostic criteria plus description of the symptoms in children's own words or the presence of two of the three supporting criteria of adults (see Table 2). Since these criteria were established for children, more children have been diagnosed with RLS, and there is a growing awareness that RLS is not especially rare in children. In fact, a recent population-based epidemiological study called the Peds REST Study noted an RLS prevalence of 2% in children between the ages of 8 and 17 years. Reports have also identified an association between iron deficiency, anemia, and childhood RLS, just as in adult RLS populations.

Table 4   Diagnostic Criteria for RLS in Children (2 to 12 Years of Age)

- The child must meet all four essential adult criteria (see Table 2)
  AND
- The child describes the symptoms in his or her own words that are consistent with leg discomfort. Examples of such words and phrases used by children include "tickle," "boo-boos," "owies," "spiders," "bugs," "want to run," and "a lot of energy in my legs."
  OR
- The child meets all four essential adult criteria
  AND
- The child meets two of the three supporting adult criteria (see Table 3).

20. My father, who is 69 years old, has been diagnosed with Alzheimer's disease. Recently, I have noticed that in the evening when lying in bed, he moves his legs and tries to get up and walk. Are these symptoms due to the nighttime agitation commonly seen in Alzheimer's disease or is he developing another movement disorder?

Nighttime agitation is very common in patients with Alzheimer's disease (AD), particularly in the advanced stages of the illness. As evening approaches, these patients will often become very agitated and anxious and begin pacing up and down. These activities may continue throughout the night. These features, which are part of what is called **"sundowning" syndrome** or **nighttime agitation syndrome**, cause severe sleep disturbances at night, often leaving patients sleepy throughout the day. Thus, this pattern represents a reversal of the normal sleep–wake rhythm. Also, in the advanced stages of AD, some patients have hallucinations (i.e., seeing, hearing, or feeling things which do not exist) and experience vivid, agitated, and fearful dreams. The sundowning or nocturnal agitation syndrome is one of the main reasons for placement of patients with AD in nursing homes or special institutions.

Symptoms such as walking, getting out of bed, and moving would suggest that the patient may have something more than sundowning or hallucinations. Rubbing the legs, trying to get up and walk, and then coming back to bed again repeatedly, when these symptoms occur in cognitively impaired patients, may suggest an additional sleep disorder such as RLS (see Question 21).

"Sundowning" syndrome (nighttime agitation syndrome)

A condition associated with Alzheimer's disease in which the sleep–wake cycle is reversed so that the person is active and agitated at night and sleepy throughout the day.

PART THREE

Symptoms and Diagnosis of Restless Legs Syndrome

Is there a laboratory test to confirm the clinical diagnosis of RLS?

Why do RLS symptoms get worse in the evening?

Is RLS a neurological disorder, a movement disorder, a sleep disorder, or a systemic disease?

More . . .

21. How do physicians diagnose RLS in elderly or cognitively impaired (demented) patients who may not be able to provide an adequate history?

Because of impairment of cognition, judgment, and memory, some patients may not be able to give adequate history to satisfy the standard four essential criteria (see Question 4) necessary to make the diagnosis of RLS. In recognition of this fact, the NIH Workshop in 2002 recommended some guidelines for diagnosing RLS in cognitively impaired subjects; these guidelines are listed in **Table 5**. In this population of patients, RLS may be aggravated by measures such as the use of restraints at night to prevent patients from wandering and the use of medications such as antipsychotic medications (dopamine blockers) and antidepressants.

Table 5   Diagnostic Criteria for Probable RLS in Cognitively Impaired Elderly Patients

Essential Criteria (All five are needed for diagnosis.)
- Evidence of leg discomfort, such as rubbing the legs and groaning while holding the legs.
- Excessive motor activity in the legs, such as pacing, fidgeting, tossing and turning in bed, cycling movements of the legs, repeated foot tapping, rubbing, and inability to remain seated.
- Evidence of leg discomfort present or worsened during periods of rest or inactivity.
- Evidence that the leg discomfort is diminished with motor activity.
- The first two criteria occur only in the evening or at night or are worse at those times.

Suggestive Criteria
- Satisfactory response to dopaminergic medications.
- Past history, obtained from a family member or a caregiver, that is suggestive of RLS.
- History of RLS in a first-degree relative (sibling, child, or parent).
- Presence of PLMS during polysomnographic recording (see Question 34).
- Significant sleep-onset problems.
- Excessive somnolence during the day rather than sleeping at night.

22. Is there a laboratory test to confirm the clinical diagnosis of RLS?

There is not a single laboratory test available that can confirm the presence of RLS (see Question 4); instead, the diagnosis is based entirely on an analysis of the patient's symptoms. There are, however, some laboratory tests whose results may give support to the clinical essential criteria, particularly in those cases with atypical features or when the patient is unable to answer all four essential diagnostic criteria questions adequately and accurately. One such test is an overnight **polysomnographic (PSG) study** (see Question 31), which may show periodic limb movements in sleep (PLMS) in at least 80% of patients with RLS (see Question 34). In approximately 20% of RLS patients, no PLMS may be noted on the first night of PSG study (see Question 30). The result of other tests, including immobilization test and actigraphy (see Question 28), may strengthen the clinical suspicion of RLS and may help determine the severity of the condition. These tests are also important for monitoring the treatment and for determining the efficacy of the drugs during the clinical drug trials.

There is not a single laboratory test available that can confirm the presence of RLS.

Polysomnographic (PSG) study

A recording of activities (physiological characteristics) from many body systems and organs during sleep at night.

23. Why do RLS symptoms get worse in the evening?

One of the fundamental characteristic features of RLS is that the symptoms are present exclusively in the evening or become worse in the evening. This is the pattern at least in the early stages of the disease; in the advanced stages of the illness, symptoms may appear earlier in the day, and in very severe cases and advanced stages, symptoms may be present throughout the day. Even in the latter cases, symptoms become worse in the evening, disturbing sleep severely. Given this pattern, one of the questions initially raised by researchers

Symptoms and Diagnosis of Restless Legs Syndrome

was whether this worsening in the evening reflects the fact that the evening is usually the time to relax and become inactive. As noted earlier, quiescence or inactivity triggers RLS symptoms.

Another factor to consider is whether RLS symptoms have a true circadian rhythm. The term "circadian" is derived from Latin: *circa* meaning "about" and *dias* meaning "day." The circadian rhythm covers slightly more than 24 hours (24.2 hours, to be precise) and is regulated by the master body clock located deep inside the brain. It is synchronized with the outside time by external light and darkness, as determined by sunrise and sunset. RLS symptoms tend to peak between approximately 9 P.M. and 4 A.M. This worsening of symptoms is due to a circadian rhythmicity, rather than just the person's inactivity during this period. Nighttime is also when the body experiences its daily increase in the level of **melatonin**, the hormone secreted by the pineal gland in the deeper part of the center of the brain (hence melatonin's nickname of "hormone of darkness"). Melatonin is a circadian marker adjusting internal and external clocks.

Melatonin

A hormone secreted by the pineal gland in the deeper part of the center of the brain at night, which serves as a circadian marker.

Some early investigations of RLS patients measuring both subjective and objective features of RLS during two days of normal sleep–wake cycles followed by 36 hours of sustained wakefulness noted that both subjective and objective measures of RLS increased in the evening and night and that these increases were not related to periods of inactivity. It was also shown that the circadian rhythm follows body temperature rhythm, such that RLS symptoms worsen with the falling phase of the body temperature rhythm, which occurs late at night and in the early morning. RLS symptoms are at a minimum in the late morning, around 10 to 11 A.M.

Moreover, as noted in the answer to Question 5, RLS symptoms are related to iron and dopamine dysfunction: Both iron and dopamine levels have a circadian rhythm, with the lowest levels being noted in the evening when the RLS symptoms are worse. Furthermore, melatonin suppresses dopamine, and this factor is partly responsible for the nocturnal peak of RLS symptoms.

24. I am a 38-year-old woman with iron-deficiency anemia. I have noticed recently that I am getting an urge to move my legs, preceded by creepy-crawly feelings in the evenings while I am trying to get to sleep. Could these symptoms be due to iron deficiency or am I developing RLS symptoms?

Iron-deficiency anemia can cause generalized symptoms of malaise, tiredness, weakness, and fatigue. Children may manifest hyperactivity and generalized restlessness as a result of iron-deficiency anemia. Also, in experimental studies in rats, iron deficiency caused generalized restlessness resembling RLS.

Clinical studies and investigations over the years have demonstrated a clear connection between iron deficiency, anemia, and RLS (see Question 5). This association was first mentioned by Karl Ekbom, who brought the entity of RLS to the forefront of the medical profession in the middle of the twentieth century. More recent studies have clearly shown an abnormality of brain iron storage in at least a subgroup of patients with idiopathic RLS. Furthermore, many conditions associated with iron deficiency, such as pregnancy, chronic kidney failure, and repeated blood donations, are associated with high prevalence of RLS.

The symptoms of an urge to move the limbs preceded by creepy-crawly sensations in the evening, therefore, are highly suggestive of RLS in a person with iron deficiency. If the person fulfills the other two essential criteria (see Question 4) of relief with movement and worsening with inactivity, then he or she will be diagnosed with RLS.

25. I was told that RLS is more common in Western countries than in Eastern countries. Is this true and, if so, why?

Many epidemiological surveys have clearly shown a prevalence of RLS of approximately 10% and a prevalence of severe RLS of 2.7% in the adult population of Western countries (North American continent and Western Europe). Studies in some Eastern countries have shown a much lower prevalence (less than 1%). Based on these studies, researchers have concluded that there is a lower prevalence of RLS in the Eastern Hemisphere. This disparity in rates may be due to some ethnic or racial differences or the presence of more frequent iron-deficiency anemia in this population. Some later studies from Japan and India, however, found a prevalence that falls in between the Eastern and Western prevalences or, in some cases, is as high as the prevalence in Western countries. This question cannot be answered definitively until further epidemiological studies from other Eastern countries have been conducted on a large scale.

26. Is RLS a neurological disorder, a movement disorder, a sleep disorder, or a systemic disease?

RLS is a neurological disorder (i.e., resulting from a functional alteration of the central or peripheral nervous system) associated with abnormal sensations and an urge to move (therefore also a movement disorder), which collectively lead to severe sleep disturbance. In that sense, it is also a sleep disorder. If future investigations demonstrate that most cases of idiopathic RLS are associated with iron deficiency or other systemic metabolic dysfunction, then RLS may be reclassified as a systemic disease resulting from a systemic biochemical abnormality. This form of the disease is found in a subgroup of patients but not in all patients, as documented by a finding of low serum **ferritin** level (ferritin is a protein that is responsible for systemic iron storage).

Ferritin

A protein in the blood that is responsible for systemic iron storage; it binds to iron in the blood.

27. Because of my RLS symptoms (which are frequent, occurring almost every night), I have severe difficulty falling asleep and staying asleep—so I do not get an adequate amount of quality sleep. Will this sleep deficit be harmful in the long term?

Sleep disturbance is not listed as an essential or supportive feature of RLS. Nevertheless, in a large survey in a primary care setting in the United States and Europe, covering more than 23,000 patients, the most troublesome symptoms (as rated by almost half of the patients) were sleep-related disturbances. In the same study, approximately 69% of those patients with moderately severe to severe idiopathic RLS (i.e., those participants who experienced RLS symptoms at least twice weekly) reported that they took more than 30 minutes to fall asleep, and 60% woke up three or more times per night. In a recent epidemiological study, those patients complaining of insomnia, who woke up in the middle of the night and had difficulty falling asleep in 15 minutes or more, complained of daytime symptoms such as lack of attention, lack of concentration, and fatigue. Many RLS patients do not complain of excessive sleepiness despite having severely disturbed sleep at night. Other patients complain of excessive sleepiness in the daytime that affects their daytime function and concentration.

Limited polysomnographic studies have been conducted in RLS patients to investigate disturbance of sleep onset and sleep duration. All of these studies have documented significant sleep disruptions in RLS subjects. Unfortunately, as yet no studies have adequately addressed the long-term consequences of such sleep disruption. Many sleep deprivation studies have noted harmful consequences in the long run following sleep disturbances, including increased cardiovascular morbidity, obesity, anxiety, depression, and decreased memory. Other experimental sleep deprivation studies in humans have convincingly demonstrated an association of short sleep duration with obesity and diabetes mellitus—both conditions that may cause increased morbidity and mortality.

An important point to consider is that a significant number of RLS patients are left with chronic insomnia despite improvement or complete resolution of their RLS symptoms. RLS patients, therefore, need to be studied for chronic sleep deprivation to understand the consequences of sleep disturbances in these conditions.

28. Is there a laboratory test to measure leg movements and assess the severity of these movements?

Periodic limb movements in sleep (PLMS)

Leg movements that occur periodically during sleep and that are characteristic of RLS.

Leg movements in RLS may include both those occurring periodically during sleep (**periodic limb movements in sleep [PLMS]**) and those occurring during relative inactivity while awake (**periodic limb movements in wakefulness [PLMW]**), which occur in most of the RLS patients. Several laboratory tests are available to measure these movements and assess their severity.

Overnight PSG will show PLMS in at least 80% of RLS patients. The PLMS index (the number of movements per hour of sleep) may indicate RLS severity and is useful for monitoring purposes. Remember, however, that PLMS are not present in the remaining 20% of patients during the first night of PSG study.

Similarly, PLMW can be measured by the **suggested immobilization test (SIT)**. In this test, the patient sits quietly on a bed with legs outstretched without moving (unless it is absolutely necessary) and without watching television, reading, or talking. Leg symptoms of sensory discomfort are monitored by questionnaire or by a visual analogue scale (VAS) every 5 to 15 minutes for quantification purposes. The VAS is a scale showing a line from 0 to 100 millimeters (mm); the patient is asked to assess the severity of symptoms from 0 to 100 (where 100 means the maximum intensity and 0 means no discomfort). In addition, leg movements are monitored by measuring the electrical activities of the muscles (electromyography [EMG]) by placing a sensor on the upper part of the tibialis anterior muscle (located in the anterior and lateral parts of the upper leg between the knee and ankle joints). By quantifying the sensory discomfort and the EMG activity (PLMW), the severity of the disease can be assessed. The test has been standardized by performing the SIT in normal healthy subjects without RLS and comparing the leg counts obtained in the controls and in the RLS patients.

Periodic limb movements in wakefulness (PLMW)

Leg movements that occur periodically during relative inactivity and that are characteristic of RLS.

Suggested immobilization test (SIT)

A test in which the patient sits quietly with legs outstretched, and leg movements are monitored to assess periodic leg movements in wakefulness (PLMW).

Symptoms and Diagnosis of Restless Legs Syndrome

An alternative way to monitor leg movements is by actigraphy, which involves wearing a watch-like device on the ankle.

Actigraphy

A test in which a motion detector is placed on the leg, and leg movements are monitored to assess periodic leg movements in sleep (PLMS).

An alternative way to monitor leg movements is by **actigraphy**, which involves wearing a watch-like device on the ankle. The actigraph is a motion detector that records leg movements and determines the number of PLMS. The data can be downloaded to a computer and analyzed. An actigraph (or actometer) measures accelerating and decelerating motions. Several actigraphs are available on the market, although not all are standardized to measure the leg movements, including PLMS, quantitatively. For clinical purposes, these devices are not very useful and are used mostly as research tools.

29. I have been diagnosed with RLS based on my symptoms and pattern of progression. Which blood tests are important for me?

As stated earlier (see Question 4), there is not a single laboratory test available whose results can definitively establish a diagnosis of RLS. Even so, certain blood tests are important especially to detect iron deficiency (see Question 24) and some comorbid conditions (or secondary causes of RLS) associated with RLS (see Question 40). Blood tests for detecting iron status may include determination of hemoglobin, total red blood cell count, serum iron level, total iron binding capacity, percentage of iron saturation, and ferritin and transferrin levels (proteins that are responsible for transport and storage of iron in the body). The prevalence of RLS is relatively high in patients with kidney failure and patients with diabetes mellitus (sugar diabetes), so other tests may include fasting blood glucose to exclude diabetes mellitus and serum creatinine and blood urea nitrogen tests to document kidney functions. Serum folate levels should also be obtained, as folic acid deficiency is sometimes associated with RLS.

30. Can RLS be diagnosed from an overnight sleep study (polysomnographic test)?

Polysomnographic (PSG) study is not routinely recommended for the diagnosis of RLS unless some associated condition (e.g., sleep apnea) is suspected. An overnight PSG study may not be enough to make a diagnosis of RLS, though its results may strengthen the clinical suspicion by documenting supporting evidence of the presence of PLMS (in 80% of RLS patients). Quantifying PLMS and identifying the PLMS index may be important in monitoring the effectiveness of treatment and for assessing the efficacy of a drug during clinical trials. Thus, although PSG may not be diagnostic for RLS, it has a definite role in this condition, particularly in atypical cases of RLS.

31. What is a PSG test?

An overnight sleep study is a recording of activities (physiological characteristics) from many body systems and organs during sleep at night. This painless procedure should not cause any discomfort to the patient. No needles are used, and the subject does not receive any electrical shock. The person having the test is connected by many sensors and wires to the equipment that records various activities. A typical recording continuously registers the electrical activities of the brain (**electroencephalogram [EEG]**), the muscles (**electromyogram [EMG]**), eye movements (**electro-oculogram [EOG]**), heart rhythm (**electrocardiogram [ECG]**), respiratory pattern, snoring, body position, and blood oxygen saturation during sleep at night.

Electrical activities of the brain (EEG) are recorded by using 3 to 10 channels of a polygraph. The polygraph

Electroencephalogram (EEG)

A recording of the electrical activity of the brain.

Electromyogram (EMG)

A recording of the electrical activity of the muscles.

Electro-oculogram (EOG)

A recording of the electrical activity associated with eye movements.

Electrocardiogram (ECG)

A recording of the heart rhythm.

is somewhat similar to the "lie detector" machine (polygraph test) used in some court cases. Of course, an overnight study takes place in the sleep laboratory, and it records many more physiological characteristics than those studied during lie detector tests.

For an EEG recording, electrodes or sensors (small, cup-shaped or flat disks measuring 5 to 6 mm in diameter) are attached with glue to the scalp; these attachments are painless. The sensors are connected by wires to the amplifiers of the polygraph. The electrical activities generated on the surface of the brain are tiny currents that must be augmented or amplified before they can be recognized on the monitor of the computer or recording paper; hence, an amplifier is an essential part of the polygraph. Most laboratories now use computers rather than voluminous amounts of recording paper for recording throughout the night.

To record eye movements (EOG), surface disks are placed over the upper corner of one eye and the lower corner of the other eye. Electrical activities of the muscles (EMG) are routinely recorded by placing sensors over the chin and outer aspects of the upper legs below the knees bilaterally. EEG, EOG, and EMG readings are used to identify the different sleep stages.

In most cases, the respiration pattern is recorded by using three channels. A sensor is placed over the upper lip, below the nose, to record air flow through the nose and mouth. In most laboratories, in addition to oronasal thermistors (air flow sensors) to record airflow through the nose and mouth, nasal pressure is recorded because this technique detects the flow limitations better than the thermistor. A band across the chest and another band across the abdomen (inductance plethysmography) register respiratory effort by recording chest and abdominal excursion during breathing. In the most common type of sleep apnea, the air flow channels recording the activities from the sensors placed below the nose show no activity or markedly reduced activity, whereas the channels registering chest and abdominal movements are deflected in opposite directions, indicating obstruction in the upper airway passage at the back of the tongue.

Blood oxygen saturation is recorded throughout the night by using a finger clip. The finger clip registers changes in the color of hemoglobin (blood pigment); the color, which is displayed on a monitor as a number (for example, 90 to 100% in a normal person), indicates blood oxygen saturation (oxygen is carried in the hemoglobin of the blood). In patients with sleep apnea, the oxygen saturation of the blood falls below 90% when the breathing (air flow) stops.

To record snoring, a small microphone is attached over the front of the neck. Body position during sleep is monitored through a position sensor over the shoulder. The degree of sleep apnea is worse when a person lies on his or her back. In a routine overnight recording, one channel is used to record electrical signals of the heartbeat (electrocardiogram) via sensors or the electrodes placed over the upper chest.

After placement of all sensors, the connecting wires are gathered into a bundle and attached to the board next to the patient. This board is then connected by wires going through the walls or the ceiling of the bedroom to the main polygraphic machine or computer in an adjacent room, where the technician will monitor a paperless recording (or the paper in the machine, if such a recording is used) and make necessary adjustments to obtain the optimal recording. If any of the electrodes (sensors and detectors) are moved, creating artifacts in the recording, the technician will enter the patient's room and reposition the sensor so that artifacts are eliminated. The technician will also watch the video if such a recording is used (most laboratories generally use simultaneous video recording to observe any abnormal movements and behavior during sleep).

The patient generally comes to the laboratory in the evening around 8:00 P.M. The technician explains the procedure to the patient and tries to set the patient at ease. Making the connections and preparations of the machine and explaining the procedure generally takes one to two hours. The technician then turns the lights off at the approximate bedtime of the particular individual and asks the person to get ready to sleep. If the patient must get up in the middle of the night to visit the bathroom, the bundle of wires can be easily disconnected from the machine and clipped to the patient's pajama or nightwear, then reconnected upon returning to bed. In the morning, the technician comes to the room around 6:00 to 7:00 A.M. to turn the lights on, remove the electrodes from the patient's skin, and clean the skin surface. The patient is then ready to go home unless he or she is scheduled to have a multiple daytime sleep study.

The severity of RLS can be determined by both clinical assessment and by using standardized scales developed for this purpose.

32. How do physicians determine the severity of RLS?

This is a very important question for the purpose of treatment and clinical drug trials. The severity of RLS can be determined by both clinical assessment and by using standardized scales developed for this purpose. Clinical assessment focuses on determining the frequency and intensity of symptoms. In other words, if the symptoms occur once a week or every other week, then the patient would be considered to have mild RLS. If symptoms occur frequently, at least two to three times per week, then the disease would be considered moderately severe. If symptoms occur every day, then it would be considered very severe. There is no measurement method to determine the intensity of symptoms except for patients' subjective reports.

It is also important to know if the symptoms occur only in the evening or if the symptoms have begun appearing in the early afternoon or later in the daytime, which may indicate either progression of the disease or augmentation (see Question 74). If the symptoms occur only during periods of forced inactivity (e.g., riding in a plane or car, or sitting for long periods while watching a movie in a theater or listening to a concert), then the disease is considered mild and intermittent. Several community studies have indicated that approximately 40% of patients have symptoms at least weekly, another 40% have less than weekly symptoms, and 20% of patients have daily or almost daily symptoms; the last subgroup suffers from severe RLS symptoms. Based on physician diagnosis reports, 2.7% of patients suffer from severe RLS.

Several scales can be used to determine the severity of RLS. The most useful scale, which is employed by all RLS specialists, is the **International RLS Study Group Rating Scale (IRLS)**. This scale measures the symptoms of RLS as well as the impact of symptoms on sleep, daytime function, and mood. The IRLS has been validated, which means that it has been proven to truly measure the severity of RLS; the evidence of its validity has come from blind assessments carried out

International RLS Study Group Rating Scale (IRLS)

The most widely used scale for identifying the severity of RLS; it measures the magnitude of RLS symptoms as well as the impact of symptoms on sleep, daytime function, and mood.

by investigators in different countries and in different clinical drug trials.

The IRLS is not used to diagnose RLS, but rather to measure its severity. The diagnosis must have been established based on the essential criteria discussed in Question 4. The IRLS includes 10 questions with 5 possible answers (ranging from 0 to 4). The maximum score is 40 and the minimum score is 0 (indicating no RLS). A score of 1 to 10 indicates mild RLS, 11 to 20 indicates moderate RLS, 21 to 30 indicates severe RLS, and 31 to 40 indicates very severe RLS. The IRLS is very useful for measuring the treatment response and as part of drug trials.

Another useful scale is the Johns Hopkins Rating Scale (JHRS), which measures the severity of RLS by the time of onset of symptoms. Other scales, which are used mostly during clinical drug trials, include the Clinical Global Impression (CGI), which is based on the physician's impression of the patient's condition, and the Patient Global Impression (PGI), which is based on the patient's assessment of his or her symptoms.

33. I am a 55-year-old man. On average, on three out of every seven nights, I experience severe leg cramps in the middle of the night that disturb my sleep. I toss and turn, and I rub my legs to get relief. What can I do? What causes the cramps?

Most people describe leg cramps as painful, crampy sensations in the legs, usually affecting the calf muscles and occurring in the middle of the night. Colloquially, these events are described as "Charlie horses." They often cause problems with sleep maintenance and may occasionally be associated with daytime sleepiness. Episodes are more common in older individuals than in younger ones. Leg cramps are usually unilateral, affecting one leg at a time.

An occasional leg cramp at night, which wakes a person from sleep once a while, may not cause much sleep disturbance and may not be associated with any significant underlying disorder. Before trying any measures to relieve the leg cramps, however, it is important to determine whether an underlying cause is present. Frequent leg cramps that occur not only during the night but also during the daytime may suggest that another disorder is at work. Therefore, the affected individual should consult a professional who will try to identify the cause of this complaint. Once a cause is found, treatment should be directed at the underlying problem, which will generally relieve the leg cramps.

Sources of leg cramps may include a variety of general medical disorders (e.g., kidney failure, low blood sodium and calcium, heart failure, arthritis, reduced function of the thyroid and parathyroid glands, diabetes mellitus), neurological disorders (e.g., amyotrophic lateral sclerosis [Lou Gehrig's disease], diseases of the nerves innervating the muscles in the legs, Parkinson's disease, muscle-related diseases), and drugs (e.g., after ingestion of lipid-lowering agents or diuretics that help produce urine). Many women also complain of cramps in the later stages of pregnancy. In addition, vigorous exercise is associated with cramps. Finally, a rare form of familial cramping exists.

Nocturnal leg cramps can sometimes mimic RLS and fulfill the four essential diagnostic criteria. Further questioning, however, will differentiate leg cramps

Nocturnal leg cramps can sometimes mimic RLS and fulfill the four essential diagnostic criteria.

from RLS. Leg cramps generally involve a single muscle and are localized and not diffuse. In RLS, by comparison, the entire lower leg is affected. Nocturnal leg cramps cause severely localized muscle pain, and the focal muscle contraction is visible as a knot; this does not happen in RLS. Also, nocturnal cramps usually last for a few minutes, whereas RLS may last for many minutes and sometimes for hours.

When all these causes are excluded, there remains a group of individuals who experience nighttime leg cramps of unknown origin. Treatment for these patients consists of both drug and nondrug therapies. Stretching and massaging the legs and bending the foot upward may help. If these nondrug treatments fail, a small dose of quinine sulfate may be administered to patients who experience disabling nocturnal cramps. Quinine is not available in the United States at present; its use has been discontinued in this country because of the serious side effects associated with this drug. In any case, pregnant women and patients with liver disease must avoid quinine.

34. My bed partner tells me that I toss and turn in bed and sometimes keep moving my legs with a regular rhythm, kicking my partner. Is this RLS?

The symptoms described here are suggestive of periodic limb movements in sleep (PLMS). In PLMS, certain kinds of movements affect mostly the legs but occasionally the arms; these movements occur in a periodic or semi-periodic manner during sleep, mostly during non-REM (rapid eye movement) sleep. The patient moves his or her legs in a periodic fashion, for perhaps an hour or so, and then stops moving. The movements recur intermittently throughout the night. During the dream stage of sleep (REM sleep), they generally stop. The bed partner may be able to describe the person's movements, which usually include bending of the toes and foot upward, sometimes bending of the knees, and occasionally bending of the arms and forearms every 20 to 40 seconds (with a range of 5 to 90 seconds).

During some of these movements, the patient may briefly wake up. Although the patient with PLMS may be unaware of this awakening, a sleep specialist can detect it by looking at the brain waves (EEG) during an overnight polysomnographic study (see Question 31). The brain wakes up briefly (3 to 14 seconds), causing the EEG to show a change from sleep to waking rhythms. If you briefly wake up in this manner repeatedly throughout the night, your sleep will not be consolidated. The resulting poor quality of sleep will lead to daytime fatigue and sleepiness. Whether PLMS causes sleep disturbance, giving rise to daytime fatigue and tiredness, remains somewhat controversial.

At least 80% of patients with RLS have PLMS. In addition, PLMS may occasionally occur as an isolated condition or be associated with a variety of other medical and neurological illnesses, medications, or primary sleep disorders. Such movements have been noted in a large percentage of patients with narcolepsy, obstructive sleep apnea syndrome, and REM behavior disorder. In particular, some antidepressant medications may aggravate these movements. Sometimes PLMS may occur in normal individuals, particularly elderly persons. In some patients with RLS, the abnormal leg movements may be noted during wakefulness (PLMW). Both PLMS and PLMW can be diagnosed from the recordings made during an overnight sleep study (see Question 31).

To ascertain whether the individual has RLS, the physician will first ask several questions to decide whether he or she meets the minimal criteria established by the International RLS study group (see Table 2) and then perform a thorough physical examination. Based on the history and physical examination, the physician with a special interest in RLS should be able to differentiate RLS from other conditions that may mimic RLS, and may be able to determine whether the RLS has a specific cause or is associated with other conditions (e.g., iron-deficiency anemia, pregnancy, kidney disease). The physician may ask for some laboratory tests to differentiate RLS from these other conditions.

35. I am a 65-year-old woman who has had RLS symptoms for many years. Recently, I have become very depressed. Can RLS cause depression?

In many community- and population-based surveys and clinical samples, depression and anxiety have been noted to be very common in patients with RLS. In this regard, it is interesting to note that Wittmack (see Question 3) described RLS-like symptoms under the heading of "anxieties tibiarum" in the nineteenth century. Similar reports are available in the contemporary literature.

In the general population, both RLS and depression are relatively common; the overall prevalence of both ranges from 5 to 10%. Patients with both conditions may have a positive family history, and females are more likely to develop these comorbidities. In some cases, the comorbidity of depression or anxiety and RLS may occur by chance, reflecting the high prevalence of both conditions in the general population. In other cases, patients suffering from RLS later develop symptoms of depression or anxiety. The symptoms of depression and anxiety may precede RLS symptoms, and it is very important to differentiate between the two because the treatment strategies for the conditions may differ. Approximately 35 to 40% of patients with RLS suffer from depression or anxiety.

One reason why patients with RLS might develop depression is that these individuals suffer from insomnia for months and years—and there is clear evidence from epidemiological studies that insomnia predisposes persons to depression. Another possibility is that the same common biochemical mechanism could be responsible for both conditions. For example, there is some evidence of a tendency toward dopamine deficiency in both patients with depression and those with RLS, although this point is conjectural and not well established for RLS.

The simple answer to this question is that RLS can cause depression but the association remains controversial. This association has important implications for treatment, because many antidepressant medications may worsen RLS. Although no systematic population-based studies have been carried out, there are many anecdotal and case series reports of worsening of RLS symptoms and particularly the leg movements at night after starting certain antidepressants (e.g., selective serotonin reuptake inhibitors [SSRIs] and certain tricyclic antidepressant [TCA] medications). When RLS symptoms worsen after antidepressant therapy is begun, patients often stop taking the medication or the physician may reduce the dosage level until RLS symptoms return to the baseline level.

How, then, should physicians handle patients with both RLS and depression? If these patients develop depression of mild to moderate severity and do not show signs of major depression with suicidal thoughts, they will first be treated with RLS medication; many patients will improve on this regimen, and their depression will lift after this treatment. If symptoms persist, then antidepressant medications that are known to have less adverse effects on RLS should be tried (see Question 81). Comorbid depression/anxiety and RLS can make RLS symptoms worse, negatively affecting the quality of life of the patient. For this reason, every attempt should be made to treat both conditions satisfactorily.

36. I have been told that some RLS symptoms (e.g., insomnia, excessive daytime sleepiness, lack of concentration) may also occur in people who suffer from major depression. How would I know that I am developing true depression? What are the specific symptoms of depression?

It is true that the symptoms of RLS and depression sometimes overlap.

It is true that the symptoms of RLS and depression sometimes overlap. For a diagnosis of major depression, the patient must experience five of nine specific symptoms listed in *DSM-IV-TR* (see **Table 6**). As seen in

Table 6   Diagnostic Criteria for Major Depression

Five of the nine symptoms must be present to warrant a diagnosis.
1. Depressed mood for most of the day and nearly every day
2. Decreased concentration
3. Insomnia or excessive sleepiness
4. Psychomotor (mental and physical) agitation or retardation
5. Significant weight loss (not dieting) or weight gain or a change in appetite
6. Fatigue or loss of energy
7. Recurrent thoughts of death or suicidal ideation
8. Feeling of worthlessness or inappropriate guilt
9. Diminished interest or pleasure in activities

Table 6, the first four symptoms associated with depression are also symptoms of RLS. It is therefore sometimes very difficult to differentiate between symptoms of major depression and symptoms of RLS-related depression.

37. My psychiatrist diagnosed comorbid depression and RLS and wants me to take some strong antidepressant medications. How should I be treated?

If you have symptoms of major depression as listed in Table 6, then it is important to determine whether these symptoms were present *before* you were diagnosed with RLS or if they came along *after* you had suffered from RLS symptoms for some time. If your symptoms of major depression preceded the development of RLS and you have not had any treatment for them, then you definitely need treatment—particularly if you have suicidal thoughts or if you have a severe impairment of quality of life. If this is an urgent situation, than you will need to take antidepressant medications (see also Questions 81 and 82). First your psychiatrist should try medications that do not worsen RLS (see Questions 81 and 82). If these medications do not work, then other strong antidepressants may be prescribed, starting with the smallest dose possible and gradually increasing the dose until the depression is relieved. At the same time, you should be treated for RLS effectively so that your RLS symptoms are under control, including any insomnia, as this sleep disturbance exacerbates depression.

If your symptoms of depression appeared after the development of your RLS symptoms, the first thing to do is to treat the RLS symptoms effectively—that therapy might also relieve the depression. If the depression persists despite adequate treatment of RLS, it needs treatment as discussed above.

38. Is RLS a real disease or is it just "disease mongering" as many have said?

Ask any patient who suffers from RLS, and he or she will tell you that it is a real disease. RLS is not a trivial disease, nor is it "disease mongering" as some people have labeled it, while declaring RLS to be a disease wholly created by the pharmaceutical industry in an effort to sell more drugs. RLS affects approximately 10% of the population, with 2.7% of the population having severe disease. In summary, RLS affects millions of people.

RLS is the most common movement disorder causing severe sleep dysfunction encountered in physicians' day-to-day practice. This disease has a severe impact on sleep and quality of life, leaving patients miserable night after night for weeks and months, and in some cases years. Some individuals spend night after night walking around and struggling to fall asleep; the next day, they may be unable to function because of lack of concentration, poor judgment, disordered thinking, sometimes excessive sleepiness, and depressed and anxious mood. Robert Yoakum, an RLS patient, has written a book that describes the frustrations and misery of many patients in terms of personal testimonials (see Question 100).

A recent genome-wide association study of RLS uncovered a biological basis for this disease, with common variants in certain genomic regions conferring more than a 50% increase in the risk of developing RLS-PLMS. Nevertheless, because there have not been any laboratory confirmatory tests of RLS, some skeptics continue to question the existence of the disease, even as they ignore the vast amount of research showing the iron–dopamine connection, the definite heritability of the disease, and the very good responses to drug therapy obtained during double-blind, placebo-controlled clinical trials in these patients. All of these observations should leave no doubt that RLS is a real disease.

Charlotte said:

In June 1983, I was awakened with what felt like a strong electrical shock coming down from the inside of my right knee and shooting down to my ankle. These shocks caused excruciating pain. When I jumped out of bed and stood up, they stopped. I went back to bed, fell asleep for about an hour or two and again was awakened by the same horrible sensations. In the morning, I noticed a large black-and-blue mark along the inside of my knee, which was swollen. I went to the emergency room and was told by the physician that I had burst a blood vessel and to rest.

The following two nights, the symptoms returned. On the fourth night, surviving on less than one hour of sleep, my left leg was similarly affected. Throughout the night, each of my legs took turns waking me up after no more than one hour of sleep. My nighttime agony and lack of sleep were affecting my performance at work. They adversely affected my entire life. The quality of my life was worsened. I was constantly exhausted. On the one hand, I could not wait to get into bed; on the other hand, I was frightened to do so. I knew symptoms would reappear as soon as I fell asleep.

I lived through years of agony and frustration. I was misdiagnosed constantly. I went from pain clinics to acupuncturists, vascular specialists, internists, neurologists, and massage therapists, and underwent epidurals and surgery (for what one physician called a blocked nerve in my leg). I was desperate. The biggest blow I encountered was when I was referred to a psychiatrist, who thought all my symptoms were related to my mother's death 43 years ago.

After more than a decade of suffering, I read about RLS in a Canadian medical journal. Finally, I recognized my condition and had the realization that all my seven siblings suffered from the same syndrome. I was fortunate enough to find a physician who specialized in RLS. Thanks to his empathy and knowledge, I am doing better. Presently, I am the Manhattan support group leader for the Restless Legs Syndrome Foundation, a nonprofit organization that aims to empower people and physicians with the basic knowledge of RLS.

39. What are some of the conditions that can mimic RLS?

Certain conditions can mimic RLS, making it difficult to differentiate them from true RLS. These conditions do not cause RLS, however. The RLS-mimicking conditions can be grouped under two broad headings: those that cause abnormal restlessness and those that are associated with discomfort or pain in the legs (see **Table 7**). The main overlapping symptoms between RLS and mimics confusing the diagnosis are discomfort at rest and an urge to move the legs.

RLS symptoms are persistent and not transient, unlike the case with some mimics.

Certain facts about RLS can help in differentiating true RLS from these mimics. RLS symptoms are persistent and not transient, unlike the case with some mimics. RLS symptoms are provoked by rest; some mimics are also provoked by rest (e.g., leg cramps), though not others (e.g., akathisia, generalized anxiety disorder). RLS symptoms are rapidly relieved by movement (some

Table 7   Conditions That Can Be Confused with Restless Legs Syndrome (Mimics)

Conditions Presenting with Excessive Restlessness
- Akathisia
- Generalized anxiety disorder
- Repetitive movements resulting from habits (habit spasms, such as leg shaking and foot tapping)
- Hypnic jerks
- Rhythmic movement disorder
- Painful legs and moving toes syndrome

Conditions Presenting with Leg Discomfort or Pain
- Nocturnal leg cramps
- Arthritis or joint problems (rheumatoid arthritis and osteoarthritis)
- Peripheral vascular disease (narrowing of the vessels, leading to insufficient blood flow to the legs during physical activities)
- Polyneuropathies (affecting the nerves associated with diabetes or other conditions causing small fiber neuropathies)
- Positional discomfort

mimics such as leg cramps and positional discomfort are also relieved by movement), whereas many mimics are not relieved by movements. RLS symptoms are not readily relieved by simple postural change, unlike positional discomfort in the legs. Restraint and confinement are extremely distressing to RLS patients. Sleep dysfunction is also very common in RLS and is frequently attributable to leg symptoms. It is very important to remember the four essential criteria (see Table 2) to differentiate RLS from the various mimics. In atypical cases, the supporting features (see Table 3) will prove helpful in making the diagnosis and differentiating RLS from mimics.

Akathisia literally means "inability to sit." Of all the mimics, akathisia is the most difficult to differentiate from RLS, particularly in advanced-stage RLS and when the RLS patient has severe augmentation. Akathisia most commonly appears after use of neuroleptics (medications that calm the nerves and are used to treat psychotic conditions). This condition is characterized by a desire to be in constant motion and an inability to sit or stand still. The inner feeling of restlessness or fidgetiness results in forced walking. The patient keeps moving, crossing and uncrossing the legs, rocking the whole body, marching in place, and constantly shifting the body position while sitting. Unlike in RLS, these movements do not follow a circadian pattern, but rather are present throughout the day. The near-constant movements do not relieve the intense urge to move in akathisia, in contrast to the relief of RLS symptoms obtained through movement.

Nocturnal leg cramps can also mimic RLS. As described in Question 33, it is sometimes difficult to differentiate this condition from RLS.

Habit spasms

Repetitive limb movements that are performed voluntarily initially, but later become habits.

Many normal people have repetitive limb movements that are performed voluntarily initially, but later become habits (**habit spasms**) and are performed subconsciously. These movements may include repetitive foot tapping, leg shaking, and rhythmic shoulder movements. Such patients do not complain of an uncomfortable sensation and do not have an urge to move.

The patient with polyneuropathy may complain of "pins and needles" sensations or the "legs going to sleep." These symptoms are present intermittently throughout the day, not just during inactivity or exclusively in the evening. The patient's history may disclose a cause for this type of neuropathy, such as diabetes mellitus, and neurological examination may show evidence of nerve damage in the legs in the form of impairment of sensation or impairment of leg muscle reflexes.

In the differential diagnosis between idiopathic RLS and the conditions mimicking RLS, it is important to look for subtle signs based on the history and physical examination that point to the correct diagnosis. In addition, laboratory tests may be performed to diagnose some of the conditions that mimic RLS.

40. What are some of the conditions that may be associated with RLS?

Many conditions are associated with RLS that are traditionally classified as "secondary." The term "secondary" implies causality, however, and it is unknown whether these conditions actually are responsible for RLS or simply trigger RLS symptoms in patients already predisposed (probably genetically) to this condition. Hence, the better term is "comorbid," meaning that these conditions are associated with RLS. **Table 8** lists these comorbid conditions. For the diagnosis of these comorbid conditions, a history, physical examination, and appropriate laboratory tests are important.

Table 8   Conditions Associated with Restless Legs Syndrome

- Polyneuropathies (conditions causing nerve damage), which may be caused by diabetes mellitus or other hereditary or familial neuropathies
- Iron deficiency, with or without anemia, caused by blood donations or internal bleeding
- Chronic kidney failure
- Pregnancy
- Parkinson's disease
- Respiratory-related diseases (e.g., chronic obstructive pulmonary disease) and sleep apnea
- Endocrine diseases (e.g., thyroid disorders)
- Resection of the stomach
- Gastrointestinal diseases (malabsorption syndrome)
- Medications, including antidepressants (see Questions 81 and 82)

Sensorimotor neuropathies

Nerve dysfunction causing sensory symptoms such as tingling and numbness and motor disturbances such as muscle weakness.

A subgroup of patients with RLS (called comorbid RLS) experience **sensorimotor neuropathies** (nerve dysfunction causing sensory symptoms such as tingling and numbness and motor disturbances such as muscle weakness), but the relationship between RLS and these entities remains uncertain. The sensory symptoms of RLS are described as deep, disagreeable, unpleasant, and often nonlocalizable discomfort (in approximately 20 to 25% of patients, these sensations are actually described as painful) without any associated impairment of sensation on physical examination. In contrast, the sensory features of polyneuropathies consist of tingling, numbness, burning, and stabbing sensations in a "stocking and glove" distribution, and impairment of sensation on physical examination. The sensory symptoms of polyneuropathies are present either intermittently or throughout the day and not necessarily worse in the evening; they generally are not relieved by movements. In approximately 20% to 25% of patients with idiopathic RLS, actual pain—rather than an intense disagreeable feeling—is a prominent symptom.

Another point to remember is that positive family history is present more often in patients with idiopathic RLS rather than in those with polyneuropathies. RLS is found more frequently in conjunction with diabetic polyneuropathy and certain hereditary neuropathies.

It is not exactly clear why some patients with polyneuropathy develop symptoms of RLS, whereas many patients do not develop RLS. Perhaps those patients who are genetically predisposed to develop RLS develop RLS symptoms in association with their polyneuropathies. The association of RLS and iron-deficiency anemia was discussed in Question 24. An increasing prevalence of RLS (20% to 50%) is noted in cases of chronic kidney failure, particularly among patients who are on dialysis. Clinically, the symptoms are similar in patients with comorbid renal (kidney) failure and RLS and patients with idiopathic RLS. Some reports have indicated that RLS symptoms sometimes disappear after kidney transplantation, suggesting some possible unknown biochemical factors may produce RLS-like symptoms in renal failure.

41. Is there an association between sleep apnea and RLS?

Before answering this question regarding the prevalence of sleep apnea in RLS, it is essential to understand what is meant by **sleep apnea**. The word "apnea" is derived from a Greek word meaning "for want of breath." Apnea—that is, cessation of breathing—occurring during sleep is called sleep apnea. Most people, particularly after the age of 50 to 60 years, stop breathing momentarily a few times during their nighttime sleep. This condition is normal and not a cause for concern. In a normal individual, this breathing cessation may occur as many as five times per hour of sleep. The breathing must stop for at least 10 seconds during sleep for it to be considered clinically significant. Sometimes breathing may not stop completely but rather be reduced by 30% to 50% of the normal breathing volume, a condition known as **hypopnea**. Like sleep apnea, hypopnea has both short-term and long-term adverse consequences.

Three types of apneas—upper airway obstructive, central, and mixed types—have been described in the literature. The most common and serious type is obstructive sleep apnea syndrome (OSAS). In this type of abnormal breathing during sleep, the passage of inhaled air becomes

Sleep apnea

Cessation of breathing occurring during sleep.

Hypopnea

A sleep disorder in which breathing may not stop completely but rather is reduced by 30 to 50% of the normal breathing volume.

Soft palate

A soft muscular tissue in the back of the roof of the mouth.

Lungs

The breathing organs responsible for maintaining normal respiration and blood oxygen at the optimal level.

Diaphragm

The main muscle of breathing, separating the lower chest from the upper abdomen.

obstructed in the region of the upper airway, most commonly at the level of the **soft palate** (a soft muscular tissue in the back of the roof of the mouth). Consequently, air does not enter the **lungs** (the breathing organs responsible for maintaining normal respiration and blood oxygen at the optimal level) and the blood oxygen level tends to fall below the normal level. The **diaphragm** (the main muscle of breathing, separating the lower chest from the upper abdomen) and other chest wall muscles keep contracting, trying to overcome the obstruction in the upper airway. The brain then sends impulses, telling the subject to wake up. The person then wakes up with a loud snore. As soon as the individual wakes up, the muscle tone in the upper airway and the tongue return to normal level. The tongue moves forward, the obstruction is relieved, and normal breathing resumes. This cycle repeats as soon as the individual returns to sleep.

In a mild case of obstructive sleep apnea, the cycle of apnea and normal breathing occurs only a few times. In severe cases, the cycle may repeat several hundred times, repeatedly reducing the blood oxygen level throughout the night and disturbing the individual's sleep. Because he or she obtains an inadequate amount of sleep, the person is sleep deprived and sleeps excessively in the daytime in an inappropriate place and under inappropriate circumstances.

In central apnea, the air flow stops at the nose and mouth, and the air does not enter the lungs. At the same time, the breathing effort by the diaphragm and other muscles of breathing stops. Central apnea is associated with a number of neurological disorders and may also be caused by long-term ingestion of opioid medications. Opioids are often prescribed to patients with severe augmentation and those with severe and refractory RLS (see Questions 76 and 80).

Mixed apnea is characterized by an initial period of central apnea, followed by a period of obstructive apnea. In the most common type of upper airway OSAS, the patient experiences many periods of mixed apneas as well as some central apneas.

Sleep apnea is more common in men than women, although its prevalence increases equally in post-menopausal women.

Why the muscle tone in the upper airway falls excessively in patients with sleep apnea, producing an obstruction in the upper airway, is not known. In many patients, the **uvula** (the small piece of soft pear-shaped structure that can be seen dangling down from the soft palate from the back of the tongue) and the soft palate are bulky and long, narrowing the upper airway passage. In children, large tonsils and **adenoids** (lymphoid tissues in the throat behind the nasal passage) may narrow the air passage, causing loud snoring and sleep apnea. The nerve cells responsible for maintaining muscle tone in the tongue and other upper airway muscles appear to transmit fewer impulses to these tissues. There is no evidence to suggest that most patients with sleep apnea have a structural defect in the nerve cells of the brain stem (the lower part of the brain). Of course, any neurological disorders (e.g., stroke, tumor, trauma, multiple sclerosis) that affect the brain stem or brain may cause sleep apnea as well.

The major nighttime symptoms of patients with sleep apnea consist of a long history of loud snoring, cessation of breathing repeatedly during sleep at night (witnessed

Uvula

The small piece of soft pear-shaped structure that can be seen dangling down from the soft palate from the back of the tongue.

Adenoids

Lymphoid tissues in the throat behind the nasal passage.

by a bed partner), and recurrent awakenings that disrupt and fragment the sleep. The most important daytime symptoms are excessive sleepiness at inappropriate times and under inappropriate circumstances, which may cause accidents and near-accidents during driving. Patients may be forgetful. Men may have impotence if they suffer from severe sleep apnea for a long time. Although most patients with apnea are obese and middle-aged or elderly, this condition can also strike thin people and can occur at a younger age. Close attention should be paid to these symptoms for making an adequate diagnosis because effective treatment will prevent the long-term adverse consequences of sleep apnea—high blood pressure, coronary arterial disease, heart failure, irregular heart rhythm, stroke, heart attacks, and impairment of short-term and long-term memory.

In terms of prevalence of sleep apnea, the most frequently quoted figure comes from research performed at the University of Wisconsin School of Medicine. This study showed that approximately 4% of men and 2% of women between the ages of 30 and 60 years have sleep apnea syndrome, which includes not only the sleep-recorded abnormalities but also the daytime symptoms. In the same study, analysis of overnight sleep recordings only showed that 24% of men and 9% of women experienced at least five episodes of apneas and hypopneas per hour.

Some limited studies have raised questions about whether prevalence of sleep apnea increases in persons with RLS. The repeated arousals that follow resumption of breathing after episodes of apnea are accompanied by periodic leg movements that resemble PLMS. These leg movements, which are called respiratory-related

PLMS, differ from true PLMS. Following treatment of OSAS, these leg movements are generally eliminated. Based on these leg movements during sleep, however, some patients are misdiagnosed as having RLS. It must be remembered that RLS is a disease of quiescence during period of relaxed wakefulness, whereas PLMS occurs during sleep and is noted in the majority of RLS patients.

Some anecdotal reports have described improvement of RLS symptoms after treatment of sleep apnea in patients with comorbid RLS and OSAS. In one study, following treatment of OSAS by continuous positive airway pressure (CPAP) titration, the patient showed improvements in both RLS- and sleep apnea-related symptoms.

In conclusion, the relationship between OSAS and RLS remains uncertain. Until large-scale epidemiological studies are performed in the general population, the true nature of this link (if it exists) cannot be stated definitively.

42. I was told that RLS is common in patients with chronic bronchitis and emphysema. Is this true?

Chronic bronchitis and emphysema are grouped under the term **chronic obstructive pulmonary disease (COPD)**. The question of an association of COPD and RLS at present remains controversial in absence of good epidemiological studies in the general population. This association was reported approximately 40 years ago. Since then, there have been scattered reports of RLS in COPD patients. It should be noted that the diagnosis of RLS was made in this population prior to the

Chronic obstructive pulmonary disease (COPD)

Chronic bronchitis and emphysema.

establishment of the generally accepted IRLSSG diagnostic criteria for RLS (see Question 4).

43. My friend who suffers from RLS tells me that this condition does not generally cause pain. Is this true?

For many years, it was believed that RLS patients complained of uncomfortable sensations in the legs causing an urge to move, but did not complain of actual pain. Since the standardized criteria were established (see Question 4), and numerous double-blind, placebo-controlled clinical trials have been undertaken over the years, investigators and sleep specialists have been increasingly evaluating large numbers of RLS patients and the perception of pain complaints has gradually changed. It is now believed that a large percentage of patients with RLS (at least 20% to 25%) complain of actual pain, if the question is appropriately framed. It is becoming clear that RLS is actually a painful disease. What the patient describes as a "disagreeable feeling" is similar to the uncomfortable painful sensations experienced by patients suffering from many central neurological disorders. These changes in perception have led to new thinking about drugs that are effective in controlling neuralgic (painful) conditions (e.g., painful diabetic neuropathies and post-herpetic neuralgia), such as certain anticonvulsants (e.g., gabapentin, pregabalin). Many RLS patients with painful leg symptoms respond satisfactorily to these medications. In the future, pain specialists might begin diagnosing and treating a large number of RLS patients.

44. What causes pain in general, and how does RLS cause pain?

The question of pain in RLS has long been neglected, as it was perceived that most of the RLS patients do not complain of pain. This understanding has recently changed (see Question 43), and it is now believed that up to 25% (or maybe even more) of RLS patients complain of actual pain rather than unpleasant sensations or discomfort in the legs.

The perception of pain has two components: (1) the sensation generated by stimulation of the pain-sensitive structures in the extremities or the trunk and (2) the subjective or emotional component of pain determined by the central processing of pain in the emotional brain (the limbic cortex). Following stimulation of the pain-sensitive structures of the periphery (skin surface), the impulses are transmitted through the peripheral nerves to the spinal cord (a long tubular structure of the central nervous system that connects to the brain stem and runs through the vertebral column). From the spinal cord, there are ascending projections to the brain stem (the base of the brain, which connects the main brain hemispheres with the spinal cord) and the **thalamus** (the main structure in the base of the brain responsible for termination of the ascending pain fibers). From the thalamus, the pain fibers project to the sensory part of the main hemisphere of the brain, where the sensation is centrally processed with the help of the **limbic cortex** (emotional brain). These ascending pain-transmitting fibers are modulated by several descending projections from several neurotransmitters and **neuromodulators** (chemicals in the brain that cause activation of the synapses of the nerve cell responsible for pain perception, memory storage, and sleep–wake regulation). These chemical pathways modulating pain include opioids (which produce analgesia), noradrenalin, and serotonin, which descend through the middle of the brain stem into the spinal cord and modulate the pain-sensitive structures in the spinal cord. Any dysfunction in these pain-transmitting structures in the peripheral or central

It is now believed that up to 25% (or maybe even more) of RLS patients complain of actual pain rather than unpleasant sensations or discomfort in the legs.

Thalamus

The main structure in the base of the brain responsible for termination of the ascending pain and other sensory fibers.

Limbic cortex

The emotional brain; it plays a central role in perception of pain.

Neuromodulators

Chemicals in the brain that cause activation of the synapses of the nerve cell responsible for pain perception, memory storage, and sleep–wake regulation.

nervous system will cause different types of pain perceived as burning sensation, stabbing or electric shock-like feelings, aching, or cramp-like feelings.

How RLS causes pain is not completely known, given that we do not fully understand the pathophysiological mechanisms underlying the sensory and motor manifestations of RLS. In one neuroimaging study (a special type of magnetic resonance imaging [MRI] study), when patients experienced the uncomfortable feelings associated with RLS, activation of the structures in the thalamus was observed. It has also been shown by special MRI study that in some patients with RLS, the thalamus is increased in size. This finding is controversial, however, and the role of thalamus and other pain-generating structures in RLS remains undetermined at present. Nevertheless, many patients with RLS—particularly those with severe cases and those with augmentation—respond to **narcotics** (central analgesic medications); this symptomatic relief is reversed after giving the patients narcotic antagonists. This relationship suggests a role for the opioid pathways in the generation of pain sensation in RLS. The question has been raised about whether this effect is due to alteration of opioid pathways or opioids acting indirectly through the dopaminergic pathways, whose dysfunction has been clearly noted in RLS patients.

Sleep disturbance in RLS (see Question 27) may partly be related to the presence of leg discomfort and pain in these patients. Pain may cause physical discomfort, leading to repeated shifting of body positions or anxiety and tension, thereby stimulating the arousal system and causing frequent awakenings during the night. All of these factors will cause sleep-onset problems and maintenance insomnia. In additional to its mechanical

Narcotics

Central analgesic (pain relief) medications.

and psychological effects (such as anxiety and tension), pain may interact with **neurotransmitters** (chemicals responsible for transmitting nerve signals) in the brain. These neurotransmitters (e.g., adrenaline, noradrenaline, serotonin, and acetylcholine) have considerable regulatory influence on the sleep–wakefulness relationship. For example, a serotonin deficiency in the brain may reduce the threshold for perception of pain, causing a person to feel pain very easily and experience sleep disturbance.

In a 1996 National Sleep Foundation Gallup survey, one-third of U.S. adults complained of sleeplessness and nighttime pain on an average of 8.5 nights per month; they slept only 4 hours and 36 minutes during those nights. It should also be noted that sleep deprivation, particularly REM-sleep deprivation, may sensitize a patient who is already suffering from pain, causing the pain to be perceived more severely. Thus REM-sleep deprivation may cause **hyperalgesia** (excessive perception of pain) in those already suffering from a painful condition. Pain may be a significant complaint in many RLS patients and disturb their sleep. As a consequence, such patients may need short-term use of sleeping medication.

Neurotransmitters
Chemicals responsible for transmitting nerve signals.

Hyperalgesia
Excessive perception of pain.

Symptoms and Diagnosis of Restless Legs Syndrome

PART FOUR

Physical and Psychological Effects of Restless Legs Syndrome

I was told that after many years of having RLS symptoms, a person may develop high blood pressure, stroke, or heart disease. Is this true and how does RLS cause these conditions?

Do RLS patients suffer from other compulsive behaviors, such as compulsive gambling, smoking, or eating?

Does RLS affect short-term and long-term memory?

More . . .

45. I was told that after many years of having RLS symptoms, a person may develop high blood pressure, stroke, or heart disease. Is this true and how does RLS cause these conditions?

Some limited studies have shown such association. One population-based study in the elderly identified an association between high blood pressure and RLS, but this finding was contradicted by later studies. A later cross-sectional study found an association between the RLS symptoms and cardiovascular disease including high blood pressure. These studies do not necessarily establish RLS as the cause of high blood pressure or other cardiovascular diseases, but do raise the possibility of such a causal relationship. Further epidemiological studies in a large number of patients, excluding all confounding factors, need to be done to establish a definitive link between RLS and high blood pressure, heart disease, or stroke.

An important confounding factor in RLS is the chronic sleep deprivation and sleep fragmentation experienced by persons with this disease. Many individuals with RLS have chronic sleep deprivation for months and years; as noted in Question 27, this kind of ongoing sleep disruption may be associated with many long-term adverse consequences, such as obesity, diabetes mellitus, high blood pressure, stroke, and heart disease. Therefore, it is not possible to determine whether high blood pressure and cardiovascular diseases in patients with RLS are due to RLS itself or to chronic sleep deprivation.

At least 80% of patients with RLS have PLMS, and it has been demonstrated that PLMS is associated with activation of the **autonomic nervous system** (the part of the nervous system responsible for controlling involuntary functions such as blood circulation and respiration). Owing to this repeated activation of the autonomic nervous system, there is repeated transient constriction of the blood vessels, which may eventually result in high blood pressure and the consequences of high blood pressure such as heart failure and stroke. Whether this happens in practice cannot be ascertained with certainty. A large number of apparently normal people also have PLMS but do not necessarily have high blood pressure or cardiovascular disease.

Autonomic nervous system

The part of the nervous system responsible for controlling involuntary functions such as blood circulation and respiration.

46. I have moderately severe RLS. I recently noticed that I have a compulsion to eat in the evening and during the night. As a result of this behavior, I have gained quite a bit of weight. Is this common in patients with RLS or do I have another condition?

Enough studies have not been conducted to definitively settle the question of whether excessive eating and drinking at night results from a compulsion or occurs out of boredom in RLS patients. Many anecdotal reports indicate that patients with RLS—particularly those with moderate to moderately severe disease—who are suffering from an uncomfortable feeling in the legs causing them to have a restless night follow a pattern of staying awake, getting out of bed, walking around, and, out of sheer boredom, eating some snacks and having beverages.

The habit of excessive eating and drinking may occur as a compulsive desire in patients who have been taking dopaminergic medications (see Question 47) for a long time. Indeed, this issue is one of the long-term

The habit of excessive eating and drinking may occur as a compulsive desire in patients who have been taking dopaminergic medications for a long time.

management problems with RLS. These patients may feel a compulsion or urge to eat and drink excessively. As a result of their excessive eating, particularly their high carbohydrate consumption, they gain weight.

The symptoms of excessive eating and drinking at night in RLS patients resulting in weight gain should be differentiated from the conditions known as sleep-related eating disorder and nocturnal eating/drinking syndrome. **Sleep-related eating disorder** is common in women between the ages of 20 to 30. In this condition, patients have recurrent episodes of eating and drinking during partial arousals from slow-wave sleep. These patients generally do not remember the episodes, but the behavior causes sleep disruption with weight gain. Affected individuals often have a history of sleep walking, and the condition can be comorbid with other sleep disorders (e.g., sleep walking, sleep apnea, narcolepsy) and ingestion of hypnotic medications such as benzodiazepines and non-benzodiazepine receptor agonists. The condition known as **nocturnal eating/drinking syndrome** is also more common in young women. The individual in this state is fully alert during the episode and can recall it the next morning. He or she wakes up repeatedly during the night to eat and drink and has insomnia. More than 50% of the total calories are consumed during the night. Often the individual experiences a craving for carbohydrates, resulting in weight gain.

47. Do RLS patients suffer from other compulsive behaviors, such as compulsive gambling, smoking, or eating?

Impulse control disorders (ICDs) include compulsive behaviors such as compulsive gambling, smoking, eating,

---

Sleep-related eating disorder

A sleep disorder in which a person has recurrent episodes of eating and drinking during partial arousals from slow-wave sleep.

Nocturnal eating/drinking syndrome

A sleep disorder in which a person wakes up repeatedly during the night to eat and drink and has insomnia, but is fully alert during the episode and can recall it the next morning.

Impulse control disorders (ICDs)

Compulsive behaviors such as compulsive gambling, smoking, eating, punding, or sexual behavior.

punding (complex, repetitive, purposeless behaviors), or sexual behavior. These disorders are described as commonly occurring in patients with Parkinson's disease (a degenerative disorder of the central nervous system that often impairs the sufferer's motor skills, speech, and posture) on long-term dopaminergic medications, but have been noted recently—albeit rarely—in RLS patients. The differences in the occurrence of ICDs in these two diseases may be due to the fact that Parkinson's disease patients require much larger doses of dopaminergic medications than RLS patients, and they have clear degeneration of the nerve cells in the basal ganglia (see also Question 12). In contrast, RLS patients require much smaller doses of dopaminergic medications, and there is no evidence of any structural lesion or loss of nerve cells in the basal ganglia in these patients.

ICDs are a set of complex behaviors caused by excessive dopamine stimulation in the limbic region of the brain (the part of the brain that controls varieties of emotions and behaviors), which activates dopamine-regulated reward centers of the brain. There have been a few isolated case reports of RLS patients on dopaminergic medication demonstrating behaviors such as compulsive gambling, compulsive eating, compulsive shopping, smoking, and hypersexuality as well as punding. These behaviors appear to be dose related: When the dosage of the dopamine agonist medication is reduced, the behaviors decrease. When the medications are stopped altogether, in most cases patients remain free of the compulsive behaviors.

The media have widely publicized the potential for dopaminergic agonist medications (e.g., pramipexole in most of the cases, but also ropinirole) to cause pathologic gambling and other compulsive behaviors

Punding

Complex, repetitive, purposeless behaviors.

Physical and Psychological Effects of Restless Legs Syndrome in RLS patients. Patients should be warned of the possibility of these compulsive behaviors, and family members and physicians should be on the lookout for such behaviors so that appropriate measures can be taken to alleviate the ICDs. If they occur, the dopamine medications need to be reduced or stopped and replaced with other treatment. Sometimes a patient is unaware of such ICDs, so physicians should keep in mind the possibility of these disorders in all patients with moderately severe to severe RLS who are on long-term dopaminergic agonist medications.

48. Is RLS associated with increasing incidence of obesity?

There have been recent reports of increased prevalence of obesity in RLS and of people with central obesity (big bellies) being predisposed to developing RLS. A study from Harvard University School of Public Health points to the importance of weight control in RLS patients. These researchers suggested that obese people may have lower dopamine receptor levels in the brain— and it is well known that RLS patients respond to dopaminergic medications. Further studies are needed to confirm this observation.

There are other reasons why RLS patients may have increasing incidence of obesity. For example, the medication side effect of ankle edema (fluid retention) may cause increasing weight gain. Moreover, chronic sleep deprivation (see Question 27) may cause many adverse consequences including increasing weight and obesity. The other theoretical possibility is that a dysfunction of the **hypothalamus** (a group of nerve cells and fibers located in the deeper part of the brain)—a center for controlling secretion of hormones, food and water intake, and sleep–wake regulation—may cause both the RLS

Hypothalamus

A group of nerve cells and fibers located in the deeper part of the brain that serves as a center for controlling secretion of hormones, food and water intake, and sleep–wake regulation.

symptoms and increasing food and water intake and weight gain. No scientific evidence has been gathered to prove this hypothesis, and it remains a matter of conjecture at present.

49. Is RLS due to a deficient or excessive amount of dopamine?

The answer to this question at present remains somewhat controversial. Dopamine deficiency is known to be the cause of Parkinson's disease. The general view is that in RLS, there is a dopamine deficiency in the basal ganglia or a relative lowering of the dopamine level in the evening. This hypothesis is based mainly on the therapeutic response noted (at least initially) in almost every patient with RLS who takes dopaminergic medications. Some neuroimaging findings suggest a deficiency of dopamine may play a causative role in RLS, though other studies have produced contradictory results. Thus indirect—but not direct—evidence suggests that there is a dopamine deficiency in RLS.

The initial report on this topic, which was published in 1982, showed an improvement of RLS symptoms after levodopa (L-dopa) ingestion. Subsequent reports indicated that even a low dose of dopamine nearly always relieves RLS symptoms. This is the basis of a diagnostic test, which involves administering L-dopa and looking for a response in reducing the RLS symptoms. The efficacy of dopaminergic treatment in RLS has been clearly established through several open-level and double-blind clinical trials. Ingestion of a dopamine antagonist will worsen RLS symptoms.

The dopamine activity in the body has a circadian rhythm, with the lowest levels of dopamine occurring in the evening. Of course, that is the time when RLS symptoms

The dopamine activity in the body has a circadian rhythm, with the lowest levels of dopamine occurring in the evening.

are noted prominently. Furthermore, iron deficiency, which may reduce the production of dopamine, also triggers RLS symptoms. In addition, the greater frequency of RLS symptoms with increasing age may be related to age-related depletion of dopaminergic neurons. All of these factors may be cited as indirect evidence in support of the dopamine deficiency theory in regard to the pathophysiology of RLS. Finally, limited post-mortem studies of RLS brain have not shown depletion of dopaminergic neurons. These findings are totally different from the dopaminergic neuron degeneration (depletion) observed in Parkinson's disease. In fact, some investigators suggest that RLS may result from a biochemical abnormality caused by excessive dopamine release in the basal ganglia. Augmentation (see Question 74), a side effect related to long-term use of dopaminergic medications, causes severe exacerbation of RLS symptoms and is thought to be due to a hyperdopaminergic state. Thus there is no convincing evidence of either a dopaminergic deficiency or an excessive dopamine release in RLS patients.

50. Can RLS be produced experimentally in animals so that we will have a better understanding of and treatment for this condition?

Several animal models of RLS are available, but none is completely satisfactory. A lesion causing damage to a special dopaminergic pathway in the nervous system projecting to the spinal cord in rats produced behavioral similarity to RLS in terms of restlessness, but this behavior lacks phenomenological similarities to the behaviors exhibited by human RLS patients. This particular dopaminergic pathway is located outside the basal ganglia and is not the pathway affected in Parkinson's disease that causes dopaminergic cell loss.

A second model was produced by feeding rats an iron-deficient diet. Although this practice produced restlessness resembling RLS-like behaviors, it was not quite similar to the behaviors of human RLS patients. A third model in mice has been produced by knocking out some special dopamine receptors that are active in the spinal cord; again, the behavior of the mice did not quite resemble human RLS patients' behavior. At present, there is no satisfactory animal model equivalent to human RLS for understanding the pathophysiology of this condition.

51. Can RLS symptoms be acute, requiring an emergency room visit? Can these symptoms be so severe as to drive someone to have suicidal thoughts?

Acute exacerbation of RLS symptoms is a notable feature of this disease that is encountered by most RLS specialists who see a large number of such patients. This exacerbation could be spontaneous, without any obvious triggers, or it could be triggered by iron deficiency, change of lifestyle (e.g., retirement and being more inactive, relative inactivity during hospitalization), use of certain medications (e.g., antihistamines, antinausea drugs, or antidepressants; see Question 82), or associated medical conditions. During these acute exacerbations, RLS symptoms become intense and frequent, may be present throughout the day, and may reach the "unbearable" point. In fact, many patients describe these symptoms as "torture." Similar severe symptoms may also occur in advanced stages of the illness due to disease progression.

There are numerous anecdotal reports of RLS patients going to the emergency room of a hospital to seek relief of these intense symptoms. Listen to Brian's description of his own experience:

Brian's comment:

I believe that I have had Restless Leg Syndrome for over 30 years. I can remember having the symptoms as a teenager, but not knowing what it was. My parents often told me that it was growing pains and that they would subside as I matured. However, when I was 30 years old, I had secured a job that required that I walk up to five miles every day. This was when RLS started to affect my sleep; I would rarely make it through the night without one or more severe episodes. As a result I found that I was unable to get a good night's sleep, and I was constantly tired. My mother who also has RLS would tell me that cheese was the cause of my leg problems. I stopped eating cheese but the RLS did not subside. I applied lotions, creams, and anything else that I thought could possibly stop the ever present feelings I had in my legs. On occasion, the RLS became RAS, Restless Arm Syndrome. On countless nights, I was unable to control both my arms as well as my legs. I had noticed over the years that my RLS became unbearable while on vacations. Because my wife and I travel, and many times a large amount of walking is required, the RLS was particularly bad. At night the bed sheets felt like sand paper against my skin.

RLS became so debilitating one night that I had to be driven to the hospital. The RLS started soon after my wife and I had finished dinner at a central New Jersey restaurant. My wife was driving because I simply could not sit still. Finally it got so bad that I got out of the car and ran the last mile to the hospital. After waiting what seemed like hours, an emergency room doctor spoke to me. To my amazement the doctor could not pinpoint what exactly was happening to me. I couldn't sit, nor could I stand in one place for more than a few seconds. Finally, after hours and hours they sent me home no better than I was when I first entered the hospital. The remainder of the night was a blur.

A few years later the exact same incident occurred. I was brought again to the emergency room and again a doctor examined me. This time, however, the physician knew what was causing my legs to jump uncontrollably but had no way to stop the problem. Finally after a few hours the doctor gave me a shot which would eventually knock me out.

As I left the ER I remember thinking that this was going to be part of my life for the rest of my life, but that was not the case. My wife who witnessed the suffering I had experienced for seventeen years began to research RLS on her own. After reading several books about the topic she kept seeing the name of a prominent doctor specializing in the treatment of RLS. Fortunately for us he had an office at a local hospital, and we made an appointment post haste. After speaking with his team, it was determined that I first take a sleep disorder test. The results were startling. It was the conclusion of the doctors that I had sleep apnea and a severe case of RLS. Tackling the RLS was the number one goal. The physician prescribed a drug called Mirapex. I was a bit skeptical because I was already taking a drug called Requip. Requip worked very well, however, the longer I took Requip, the more it seemed I needed to increase the dosage. I have been taking Mirapex for over a year and I have not had to increase the dosage.

My thanks go out to the physician and his team who gave me my life back.

Many patients who have experienced these unbearable symptoms affecting sleep and mood night after night have had suicidal thoughts on certain occasions, particularly those with severe depression (see Question 82). There are, however, no adequate scientific studies to verify these anecdotal reports of suicidal thoughts and desperate measures undertaken to relieve these symptoms in the occasional patient. There is one report attesting to the potential for injury in patients with uncontrolled RLS. In this case, an elderly woman with uncontrollable RLS spent most of the night standing and walking. On several occasions, she fell and sustained occasional bone fractures. Another report involves an elderly woman with RLS who was admitted to the hospital on an emergency basis with severe pain in her legs, which was relieved dramatically by use of epidural (outside the lining covering the spinal cord) morphine (a very strong narcotic).

The utter frustration and desperation of many patients with RLS are vividly described as personal testimonials in a book published in 2006: *Restless Legs Syndrome: Relief and Hope for Sleepless Victims of a Hidden Epidemic* by Robert Yoakum. Yoakum is a victim of this miserable disease himself (see Question 100).

52. Does RLS affect short-term and long-term memory?

Sophisticated neuropsychological investigations over the last two decades have clearly shown a relationship between sleep and memory. Sleep is a necessity for memory consolidation and processing. A strange fact is that most people find it easy to remember previously learned information after a good night's sleep, and our memory and concentration seem to be affected after severe sleep deprivation. RLS patients suffer from sleep deprivation night after night, for months and years. Because of this long-term sleep fragmentation and deprivation, they often experience a lack of concentration, impairment of daytime function, anxiety, irritability, and impairment of memory.

Sleep is a necessity for memory consolidation and processing.

This aspect of RLS has been largely neglected by researchers, except for two recent reports from Johns Hopkins Medical Center. In these brief preliminary studies, RLS patients were found to have impairment in some aspect of neuropsychological tests that could be ascribed to sleep disruption. Recently, a sophisticated magnetic brain stimulation study showed evidence of impairment of long-term potentiation (retention of long-term memory) in RLS patients. In a brief report from the Mayo Clinic in Scottsdale, Arizona, however, researchers noted that there was no cognitive dysfunction in older individuals with mild RLS. Further studies in large numbers of patients from different centers are needed to address this problem.

53. As I am about to fall asleep, I get electric shock-like feelings in my legs immediately followed by jerking movements. Do I have RLS or periodic limb movements in sleep?

If you have only momentary electric shock-like feelings followed by jerking movements at sleep onset without any urge to move or relief from the symptoms by movement, then you do not fulfill the essential criteria for diagnosis of RLS (see Question 4). The RLS symptoms of leg discomfort with an urge to move occur during inactivity while you are lying in bed. These symptoms last more than a few seconds and generally last for several minutes, although severe cases can last for hours. The symptoms described in this question do not fulfill the criteria for periodic limb movements in sleep (see Question 34). PLMS occurs during sleep and not at sleep onset, though PLMW can occur during relaxed wakefulness as a person is trying to get to sleep.

The symptoms described in this question resemble a condition known as **hypnic jerks**, a normal physiological phenomenon that affects as much as 70% of the general population. These sudden jerking movements of the legs and the whole body last for a few seconds and

Hypnic jerks

A normal physiological phenomenon characterized by sudden jerking movements of the legs and the whole body that last for a few seconds and always occur at the moment of falling asleep.

always occur at the moment of falling asleep. They are not accompanied by any loss of control of the urinary bladder or tongue biting, so they are not consistent with a diagnosis of nocturnal seizures. The jerking movements generally do not interfere with sleep, although sometimes repeated intense jerking movements may cause anxiety that leads to difficulty falling asleep. Similar movements may sometimes occur after waking up in the middle of the night and going back to sleep. Again, these episodes take place at the moment of sleep onset. Occasionally, the jerking movements may be accompanied by a sensation of falling or other sensory symptoms. Hypnic jerks may occur following a period of stress, fatigue, or sleep deprivation. The only treatment required is an explanation with reassurance.

54. My husband keeps tapping his feet on the ground, and sometimes he rhythmically shakes his legs whenever he is relaxing in a chair. He has restlessness of his legs. Does he have RLS?

Most likely the husband does not have RLS but further history is needed to find out if he fulfills all four essential diagnostic criteria for RLS (see Question 4). Many normal individuals, out of sheer boredom or anxiety, become fidgety and keep tapping the feet on the ground, sometimes rhythmically shaking the legs whenever relaxed in a chair. Superficially, this behavior may resemble RLS symptoms. These individuals do not have an urge to move the legs, however, and they do not have the uncomfortable sensation preceding the urge. If they are asked to stop, they can do so; then they will resume again when they are bored or anxious. Such behavior is just a kind of a habit for the individual. There is also no circadian pattern to the behavior; that is, the symptoms are not present exclusively in the evening and do not get worse in the evening. Taking into consideration all four essential criteria for RLS diagnosis, it is easy to differentiate this habit spasm from symptoms of RLS.

55. Sometimes I get "pins and needles" and tingling feelings in my legs after crossing them while relaxing. Is this RLS?

This is a very common story and does not necessarily indicate RLS. "Pins and needles" sensations as a result of temporary compression of the superficial nerves in the legs are commonly observed in many individuals after crossing the legs. These symptoms disappear upon changing the position of the legs within a few minutes. This condition is totally different from the symptoms of RLS, which include uncomfortable feelings and the urge to move the legs, with relief obtained after moving. On some occasions, however, these sensations mimic very closely RLS because of the temporary nature of the symptoms, because of the uncomfortable feelings, and because of the relief of symptoms after moving or changing the position of the legs—which fulfill three of the four RLS criteria. Such individuals do not have any circadian component to their symptoms, however. A similar phenomenon may occur after waking up from sleep in a bad posture that has caused temporary compression of a superficial nerve.

56. I am a 55-year-old woman with generalized aches and pains. I feel fatigued all day. I also have intense discomfort in my legs, with an urge to move while trying to sleep. Do I suffer from RLS, fibromyalgia, or chronic fatigue syndrome?

Any of these three conditions could be responsible for this patient's symptoms, and a detailed analysis of the symptoms is needed to arrive at the correct diagnosis.

Both fibromyalgia and chronic fatigue syndrome can cause nighttime sleep disturbance, daytime fatigue, tiredness, and sleepiness. These two conditions may occur either together or separately.

Fibromyalgia

A type of rheumatic disease that does not affect the bones or joints; characterized by diffuse muscle aches and pains throughout the body.

An estimated 3 to 6 million Americans are believed to suffer from **fibromyalgia**, a type of rheumatic disease that does not affect the bones or joints. Individuals suffering from this condition complain of diffuse muscle aches and pains throughout the body, but most commonly in the neck, shoulders, lower back, and buttocks. No single diagnostic laboratory test can detect fibromyalgia. Instead, the condition is diagnosed based on history and physical examination and after exclusion of other muscle, bone, and joint pains. A set of formal diagnostic criteria have been established for fibromyalgia that include widespread pain lasting for at least three months and tender points in at least 11 of 18 anatomically defined sites after applying finger pressure of certain minimum force. The cause of fibromyalgia remains undetermined.

Sleep complaints are very common with fibromyalgia, with patients experiencing repeated awakenings and decreased amount of total sleep. Sleep is not restorative or refreshing. As a result of the nighttime sleep disturbance, patients complain of daytime fatigue and sleepiness. Some patients with fibromyalgia also experience repeated leg jerking during sleep at night (periodic limb movements in sleep; see Question 34).

There is an increasing prevalence of RLS in fibromyalgia.

There is an increasing prevalence of RLS in fibromyalgia. Thus these two conditions could be comorbid and need to be diagnosed separately based on the essential criteria of RLS (see Question 4) and the criteria for fibromyalgia.

Fibromyalgia and **chronic fatigue syndrome (CFS)** share some overlapping symptoms. Both conditions remain controversial and have undetermined causes. Many patients with CFS report nighttime sleep disturbance, daytime fatigue, and sleepiness, similar to the symptoms noted in fibromyalgia patients. Both fibromyalgia and CFS may have comorbid sleep disorders such as RLS and PLMS. CFS is a complex and debilitating illness. Patients complain of profound fatigue, which causes them to function below their usual level of energy; this fatigue is not improved by bed rest. CFS affects more than 1 million people in the United States and is more common in women than men. An international panel of experts established diagnostic criteria for CFS, which include severe chronic fatigue for six months or longer, absence of other medical conditions explaining chronic fatigue, and presence of four or more of the following features: impairment of short-term memory or concentration; sore throat; tender lymph nodes; muscle pain; multiple joint pain without swelling or tenderness; headache different from any previous headaches; unrefreshing sleep; and post-exertional malaise lasting longer than 24 hours.

Chronic fatigue syndrome (CFS)

A complex and debilitating illness in which patients complain of profound fatigue that is not improved by bed rest.

57. My toes and feet keep moving on their own. I cannot control these movements. These movements are painful (sometimes painless) and occur all day long, while I am both resting and walking. Do I have RLS?

These symptoms do not seem to be consistent with the diagnosis of RLS. Painful or painless movements of the toes and feet present throughout the day, while both resting and walking, differ from the symptoms of RLS. RLS symptoms are present exclusively in the evening or worsen in the evening and occur only while resting,

Physical and Psychological Effects of Restless Legs Syndrome

but are relieved by walking or other movements. Also, RLS patients have a desire to move the limbs generally associated with the uncomfortable feelings. The movements described in this question are not associated with an urge to move, and they do appear not to be under the person's voluntary control. The movements of RLS are under voluntary control except in some cases, particularly in moderately severe to severe disease, where the movements could be brief and rapid, like a muscle jerk without any voluntary control.

The movements described in this question are consistent with a condition known as painful or painless legs and moving toes syndrome. This entity was first described in 1971. This condition is relatively easy to differentiate from RLS. It could be due to a dysfunction in the central or peripheral nervous system.

58. I have RLS but I do not have a positive family history of RLS, nor do I have any systemic disease (e.g., anemia, kidney failure, rheumatoid arthritis). Could my RLS be due to any environmental factor?

The cause of RLS is not exactly known. Many patients have a positive family history with affected first-degree relatives, but not all patients have a relative with RLS. When RLS is thought to result from or be associated with a disease, it is called secondary or comorbid RLS. When no associated condition is noted, it is called idiopathic or primary RLS. Idiopathic RLS most likely results from a combination of familial and environmental factors, although the nature of the environmental influences is currently unknown. In persons who do not have any genetic predisposition to the disease, it is possible that some as yet unknown environmental factor might cause a biochemical abnormality (not identified at present) in the brain that produces RLS. Even in those individuals with a positive family history, an unknown environmental factor may be responsible for triggering the onset of RLS. These family members were raised in the same environment, in the same geographical area, drinking the same water and eating similar food, and growing up in the same latitude and climate. The difference in prevalence in different regions around the world could be determined by this unknown environmental influence. Unfortunately, this aspect of RLS research has so far been neglected.

59. Is RLS a disorder of the main brain hemisphere, brainstem (the portion of the brain below the main brain hemisphere), or spinal cord (a tubular structure descending from the brainstem and connected to the peripheral [e.g., nerve roots or nerves going to the limbs] nervous system)?

None of the physiological, neuroimaging, or biochemical studies have pinpointed the exact site of origin for RLS symptoms. Changes have been noted at all levels of the central nervous system (CNS), from the spinal cord to the cerebral cortex, and there is even some evidence in some patients of possible changes outside the CNS. In the **peripheral nervous system** (the part of the nervous system that lies outside the central nervous system), physiologic studies have shown that nerve impulses are conducted normally in RLS patients. Also, there are no structural alterations in most patients, except some minor changes in the skin nerves in occasional patients. The prevalence of RLS is slightly higher in those with peripheral neuropathy (damage to the peripheral nerves).

Peripheral nervous system

The part of the nervous system that lies outside the central nervous system.

In the spinal cord, some physiological studies show evidence of increased excitability of spinal reflexes, which is thought to occur secondary to loss of inhibition as a result of dysfunction of the nervous system above the spinal cord. Physiological studies have shown evidence of increased excitability of some brain stem reflexes in RLS patients, albeit not consistently across all studies. In addition, functional neuroimaging studies have pointed to some abnormality in the upper brain stem and thalamus (a structure below the main brain hemisphere that is responsible for integration of the sensation of the body). Sophisticated neurophysiologic studies have shown changes in the sensorimotor cortex (the part of the main hemisphere that is responsible for integration of body sensation with the motor functions). Other neuroimaging studies have identified minor abnormalities in the basal ganglia (groups of nerve cells and fibers at the base of the brain below the main hemisphere), but no structural loss of nerve cells. Moreover, brain imaging studies have shown problems with iron acquisition and storage in the basal ganglia (see Question 5).

RLS is associated with minor alterations at all levels of the nervous system without any evidence of nerve cell loss.

In summary, RLS is associated with minor alterations at all levels of the nervous system without any evidence of nerve cell loss. These findings suggest a functional abnormality of the CNS, probably resulting from some biochemical abnormality (in some patients, related to the brain's iron storage problem). It appears that multiple neurotransmitters (chemicals responsible for transmission of impulses between different nerve cells and fibers) and complex interactions of CNS nerve cell networks are responsible for RLS symptoms.

60. Is RLS common in patients with chronic bowel disorders?

To date, no large-scale study has addressed this issue. Mostly there are anecdotal reports suggestive of a relationship between RLS and chronic bowel disorders, plus a few cases reported mainly from one major medical center about this proposed association. In these studies, there is an increased prevalence of RLS in patients with irritable bowel syndrome (a functional gastrointestinal disorder), Crohn's disease (an inflammatory bowel disease), and celiac disease (which causes malabsorption due to gluten sensitivity). Gluten is a protein found in wheat, barley, and rye; gluten sensitivity in some individuals is the result of an inherited autoimmune disease. Following a gluten-free diet, the bowel condition improves, and RLS also is found to be improved in some (but not all) of the patients. In Crohn's disease, RLS incidence is thought to be related to iron deficiency, which is also common in Crohn's disease and irritable bowel syndrome. An overgrowth of intestinal bacteria is found in many of these patients, who often respond to antibiotic treatment.

In summary, the association between RLS and chronic bowel disorders has not been firmly established. It is possible that some patients with these conditions are genetically predisposed to develop RLS, so that the onset of these chronic bowel disorders just triggers the RLS.

61. Is RLS a benign condition (as most people think) or is it a serious disorder (as most RLS specialists think) causing significant morbidity (impaired quality of life and suffering) and increased mortality with reduced longevity?

RLS is not a mild condition (though it may have been in the beginning, many years before the patient consulted a physician) or a trivial disease. Approximately 2.7% of the population (millions of people) suffer from severe disease posing a serious clinical challenge. In the most severe cases, symptoms may present for most of the day.

Symptoms of RLS are very frustrating to patients, many of whom think it is the worst disease they ever had. One of the most important complaints, which often prompts the patient to seek a physician's advice, is sleep disruption as a result of leg discomfort and an urge to move the legs; this problem may prevent the person from falling asleep and staying asleep throughout the night. As a result of the sleep disruption, a host of other complaints may arise, such as daytime fatigue, sleepiness, lack of concentration, memory impairment, anxiety, and depression. RLS symptoms have severe impacts on job performance, social interactions with bed partners, and family relationships. As a result of these symptoms, the patient is seriously disabled. Secondary to sleep disruption, in the long run patients may develop high blood pressure, diabetes mellitus, and severe cardiovascular disease, leading to increased morbidity (impaired quality of life and suffering) and even mortality.

RLS is a serious condition with severe short- and long-term consequences. It is not "disease mongering," and it is not a creation of the pharmaceutical industry in an attempt to sell more drugs. RLS is a real disease. Unfortunately, we do not know its cause and there is not a single diagnostic test to prove its presence, which may give the false impression that it is a psychosomatic disease.

62. Is there a difference in early-onset and late-onset RLS in terms of the clinical presentation or the natural progression of the disease?

Studies have shown clear differences between early-onset RLS (before the age of 35 to 45 years) and late-onset RLS (after the age of 45 years), but exceptions do occur. Early-onset RLS is more consistently associated with a positive family history (i.e., these patients have more affected relatives) than late-onset disease. Early-onset

RLS also has a more slowly progressive course and a longer duration of disease than the late-onset variation. In late-onset RLS, the disease progresses relatively rapidly and generally patients seek medical advice within 5 years of onset of symptoms. Late-onset RLS is frequently symptomatic or comorbid with other conditions, whereas early-onset disease is primarily idiopathic (cause unknown and not associated with any other disease). In early-onset RLS, there is greater deficiency in brain's iron storage than in late-onset RLS. Finally, in early-onset RLS, ferritin levels in the **cerebrospinal fluid** (the fluid bathing the central nervous system) are lower than in late-onset RLS.

Cerebrospinal fluid
The fluid bathing the brain and the spinal cord.

63. Why is there a delay (sometimes lasting 20 to 30 years) in making a definitive diagnosis of RLS?

In the early stage of the disease, symptoms are mild in intensity and frequency, occurring perhaps one to two times per month, with long periods of remission in between episodes. Patients, therefore, do not bother to discuss their discomfort with their physicians. Even when the symptoms become more frequent and intense, patients may hesitate to consult a physician because they are apprehensive that the condition will be labeled as psychosomatic disorder ("It's all in your head and there is nothing wrong with you"). Even now, many physicians are not aware of RLS, or they may not think it is a real condition and may find the symptoms amusing and readily label the patient as "psychoneurotic." All of these factors account for the delay in diagnosis.

Despite intense efforts by the RLS Foundation and other sleep organizations, this condition remains underdiagnosed and often goes completely undiagnosed because of the ignorance of many physicians. Most patients generally present to their physicians for relief of their RLS symptoms 20 to 30 years after initial onset of the symptoms. Collectively, the mild symptoms in the beginning of the disease course, the slow progression of the disease, apprehension about being labeled a neurotic, and ignorance about the condition are the factors driving the delay in diagnosis and treatment of RLS.

64. I have RLS. I can cope with the disease at the present time by taking medication and using some nondrug measures. How will RLS affect my quality of life over the long term?

A survey of many thousands of patients in the primary care setting (i.e., patients seen by family physicians) in several regions in Europe and the United States clearly showed a negative impact of RLS symptoms on quality of life: 64% of survey participants reported that RLS had at least some negative impact on the quality of life, and 36% reported a severe negative impact from the disease. Other surveys using quality of life questionnaires have found that RLS symptoms affect quality of life more severely than diabetes mellitus and osteoarthritis, and with equal severity as depression. Recent studies, including cross-sectional studies, have indicated that untreated RLS may severely impact the individual's general health, including his or her cardiovascular health, over the long term.

65. Are RLS patients more prone to have anemia or iron deficiency, or are they more sensitive to low iron levels in the body or the brain?

This is a very important question for which a clear answer is not available at the present time. In a subgroup of patients with idiopathic RLS, iron deficiency has been identified (either by estimating serum iron or serum ferritin levels); in these patients, giving iron supplementation along with vitamin C to promote its absorption will help alleviate both the deficiency and the RLS. In the vast majority of patients, however, iron deficiency has not been noted. In addition, some limited studies using iron supplementation in all RLS patients (not just those with an iron deficiency) have not shown any benefit related to symptoms after this treatment.

Some studies of the brain using neuroimaging techniques and postmortem examination of the brain in a few cases of RLS patients have shown reduced storage of iron in certain parts of the brain. Levels of iron, including ferritin (which carries iron for storage), in the blood of some patients with RLS may be normal, even while ferritin levels may be low in the cerebrospinal fluid (the fluid bathing the brain and spinal cord). In these patients, supplemental iron treatment will be beneficial. It is also possible that some RLS patients are more sensitive to relatively low iron levels (although within normal limits) and may experience dopamine dysfunction through the iron–dopamine connection (see Question 5). This last hypothesis is a pure speculation at present, and there are no scientific data to prove it.

PART FIVE

Treatment of Restless Legs Syndrome

How does the RLS specialist decide on treating a patient, including whom to treat and when to treat?

What are some of the medications found to be useful for RLS?

What can I do for my sleep problem associated with my RLS symptoms? Should I take sleeping medications in addition to RLS drugs?

More . . .

66. Is there research trying to advance our understanding of the genetics of RLS (e.g., identification of genes or gene products that will eventually advance therapy)?

Considerable progress has recently been made in understanding the genetics of RLS. Based on studies of case series, it is clearly established that more than 60% of RLS patients are aware of affected relatives. Genes are protein products, and investigators have begun analyzing deoxyribose nucleic acid (DNA), an amino acid in the chromosomes, as a potential source of this disease. Humans have 22 pairs of chromosomes, each consisting of paired DNA strands residing in the cell nucleus. DNA analysis is often able to identify genetic similarities between several members of a family. Using this technique, a linkage between a particular gene and RLS has been uncovered in at least five regions of chromosomes, although the genes responsible for RLS have not been found yet. Recently, two very important studies looked at genome-wide associations in RLS and uncovered common variants in certain regions conferring a more than 50% increased risk for RLS-PLMS. These findings suggest a biological basis for the RLS; it is a real disease (see Question 38). Association studies have also shown an increased risk of PLMS in persons with decreased serum ferritin.

67. Do mild cases of RLS remain mild, or do they inevitably progress to become moderate or severe? In other words, what are the natural history and course of RLS?

RLS is a chronic progressive disease. Symptoms are generally mild at onset, beginning mostly in childhood (during the history-taking process, patients will often tell their physicians that their symptoms began in childhood).

Over time, symptoms gradually increase in frequency and intensity. By the time symptoms are severe and frequent enough to affect the quality of life, the disease has often progressed for 20 to 30 years, so that the patient presents to the physician in middle age. There are certain differences in the course, however, depending on whether the illness has an early or late onset (see Question 62).

We do not know the exact natural history of the disease because there have not been adequate longitudinal studies of untreated patients to understand the natural course of the illness. It appears that the disease progresses slowly up to the age of 80 years or so; for some unknown reason, the disease then stops progressing. Patients may periodically experience remissions, in some cases lasting for weeks and months.

Patients may periodically experience remissions, in some cases lasting for weeks and months.

An interesting phenomenon is that spontaneous exacerbation of symptoms (see Question 51) may occur even when patients have been on RLS medication. These "breakthrough" symptoms may be triggered by factors such as iron deficiency, change of lifestyle (e.g., semi-retirement with increased periods of inactivity), associated medical disorders, and use of certain medications (see Question 82).

68. My family physician thought I might have RLS and referred me to an RLS specialist. Should I be treated now with drugs, which may have side effects, or should I wait to begin treatment? When should I be treated?

These are very important questions. The family physician is correct in referring the patient to an RLS specialist to make a decision regarding treatment. The choice of therapy will depend on confirmation of the diagnosis and determination of the frequency and severity of the symptoms. The diagnosis first must be confirmed based on the essential diagnostic criteria (see Question 4). If the symptoms are very mild, occurring occasionally without bothering the patient too much and not interfering with sleep or daytime function, then most likely treatment is not needed. If the symptoms, although mild, are bothering the patient or interfering with sleep, then it is worth treating the RLS. In such a case, medication may not be prescribed, but rather nonpharmacologic therapy will be recommended (see Question 70). If symptoms occur only in certain situations (e.g., watching a movie in the evening, during a long plane trip or a long drive) and those RLS symptoms bother the patient, treatment during those specific situations may be recommended. Under these circumstances, it is best to treat RLS with quick-acting medications (see Question 71). The decision to treat with medications will be decided by the physician after making the diagnosis and discussing the level of functional impairment with the patient.

69. How does the RLS specialist decide on treating a patient, including whom to treat and when to treat?

The RLS specialist will first confirm the diagnosis that the family physician suspected. This diagnosis will be based on a detailed history and the four essential criteria (see Question 4). A diagnosis must be definitively established first before any form of treatment is considered. The specialist physician will then decide if the patient has primary RLS or comorbid (secondary) RLS. This distinction is important because the comorbid conditions must be identified and treated. The next step for the physician is to determine if the symptoms are mild or intermittent without significant disability, which affects whether drug treatment will be prescribed or whether nonpharmacologic measures will be sufficient. The physician then determines the severity of RLS (see Question 32). After attending to these general guidelines, the physician will suggest the correct course of treatment.

70. Are nonpharmacologic measures helpful for RLS?

Nonpharmacologic (nondrug) measures should be followed by all patients with RLS, whether their disease is mild, moderate, moderately severe, or severe and intractable. These measures may be the only responses needed for persons who suffer from intermittent RLS characterized by infrequent (once or twice per month or once per week), very mild symptoms that are a little bit of a nuisance but do not interfere with sleep or other functions. These measures will be able to control mild symptoms in most of the cases. Some patients, however, are bothered by even these mild symptoms; they will need medication in addition to nondrug measures. Mild or intermittent RLS symptoms that occur under other circumstances, such as while going on a long trip in a plane or car, or during periods of prolonged immobility such as watching a movie in the evening, may require temporarily short-acting medications, such as a small dose of levodopa or opiates (see Question 71).

Table 9 lists the various nonpharmacologic measures. These measures are based on expert evidence and patients' histories (anecdotal evidence), rather than on rigorous scientific evidence.

Sleep hygiene measures are common-sense measures that promote and consolidate sleep and regulate the

Treatment of Restless Legs Syndrome

Table 9   Nonpharmacologic Treatment of Restless Legs Syndrome

- Follow sleep hygiene measures: Keep a regular sleep–wake schedule including weekends; sleep the amount needed to feel rested; avoid napping during the daytime; do not watch television, listen to loud music, or plan the next day's activities while in bed; adjust the bedroom environment; do not go to bed hungry.
- Consider discontinuing or reducing medications that can worsen RLS, such as antidepressants, antihistamines, and antinausea drugs (see Questions 81 and 82).
- Avoid circumstances that may trigger RLS systems, such as drinking alcohol, smoking, and consuming caffeine-containing beverages.
- Exercise regularly (mild to moderate exercise but avoid vigorous exercise, which may exacerbate RLS symptoms).
- Participate in mentally alerting activities.
- Use counter-stimulation measures.
- Participate in patient support groups.
- Take iron replacement therapy if needed as per the physician's advice.

sleep schedule, thereby avoiding the sleep deprivation that may be counterproductive to RLS. Many medications provoke RLS symptoms and, therefore, should be avoided if possible (see Questions 81 and 82).

It is best for RLS patients to avoid caffeine and caffeine-containing beverages, alcohol, and smoking as well.

It is best for RLS patients to avoid caffeine and caffeine-containing beverages, alcohol, and smoking as well. This advice is predominantly based on patients' reports. One report states that caffeinism is the cause of RLS and that avoiding this substance will prevent RLS. This is not always true, however. Even so, most RLS patients find that avoiding caffeine helps their symptoms.

It is also best for people with RLS to avoid alcohol. Its consumption may promote sleep in the evening, but when the level falls off, the person may experience repeated awakenings, disturbing sleep, and the RLS symptoms may reemerge at that time (in the middle of the night).

Some case reports indicate that smoking cessation has the ability to stop RLS symptoms; later epidemiological studies have produced contradictory results on this issue. Because some evidence in epidemiological surveys suggests that smoking might aggravate symptoms, it is best to avoid smoking. In any case, smoking has other undesirable side effects besides exacerbating RLS symptoms.

Regular exercise is helpful for promoting sleep and relieving RLS symptoms. Vigorous exercise, however, will exacerbate RLS symptoms and should be avoided. Most patients find that mental distraction or mentally alerting activities will benefit RLS symptoms. Examples of mentally alerting activities include playing video games, knitting, engaging in interesting and exciting discussions, listening to music, reading an interesting book, playing cards, and working on crossword puzzles.

Almost all RLS patients use counter-stimulation measures to relieve their symptoms, which arise mostly in the legs but sometimes in the arms. These measures include rubbing or massaging and foot massage, using a vibrator, taking a cold or hot bath or shower, leg wrapping, bicycling in the bedroom, and marching in place. Sexual activity and orgasm help many patients; in some patients, however, these activities worsen RLS.

An important nonpharmacologic measure is correcting any iron deficiency with supplemental iron if needed (e.g., if the patient's serum iron or ferritin levels are low). This decision should be made in consultation with the physician. It is not advisable to take iron replacement therapy without knowing the levels of ferritin or serum iron, as iron overload may cause serious problems such as hemochromatosis—a serious condition caused by iron deposition in the liver, brain, and other organs.

Treatment of Restless Legs Syndrome

Finally, it is a good idea for patients to join an RLS support group. In these groups, patients with RLS symptoms of different frequency and intensity get together to discuss their problems. Such meetings are a good source of education and a good way to avoid the loneliness and isolation that often occur after years of intense suffering and frustration.

71. What are some of the medications found to be useful for RLS?

Four groups of medications have been found to be useful for RLS: dopaminergic medications (agents promoting the function of dopamine, a chemical found to be deficient in patients with Parkinson's disease); anticonvulsants (drugs used to treat epilepsy); opioids (synthetic morphine derivatives used as painkillers); and sedatives-hypnotics. All of these medications must be prescribed and monitored by physicians (including RLS specialists).

Dopaminergic medication is considered the first line of drug treatment for RLS. These agents have long been used to treat Parkinson's disease and are effective in RLS, albeit using a much lower dose than that used to treat Parkinson's disease. Only two of these agents—pramipexole (brand name: Mirapex) and roprinirole (brand name: Requip)—are officially approved for use in the United States and Europe for treating patients with moderate to severe RLS. Levodopa was the first dopaminergic medication used in RLS. Levodopa by itself is inactive but is converted in the blood into dopamine, which is an active neurotransmitter. Because of levodopa's less than ideal side-effect profile, which includes a tendency to cause augmentation (see Questions 73 and 74), dopamine agonists acting directly on dopamine receptors substituting for dopamine are the preferred agents for treating RLS.

Dopamine agonists begin to act $1^1/_2$ to 2 hours after ingestion, and the action lasts for about 6 to 8 hours. By comparison, levodopa begins to act within 15 to 30 minutes, and its effects last from 2 to 3 hours. Long-acting dopamine agonists—cabergoline and rotigotine patch—have sustained action for 24 hours or longer and are thought to have a lower tendency to produce augmentation. These two drugs, however, are approved only for Parkinson's disease and not for RLS. Another dopaminergic drug, pergolide, which has been studied extensively and found to be useful in RLS, is no longer used for this disease because of its serious side effects.

There is great individual variation in responses to the various dopaminergic medications: Some patients may respond to one dopamine agonist drug but not to others. The physician will determine the best drug by trial and error.

Anticonvulsant medications have not been formally approved by the FDA for RLS but have been used successfully in some patients with this disease. These agents include gabapentin (Neurontin) and related drugs such as pregabalin (Lyrica), as well as other anticonvulsants such as carbamazepine (Tegretol), oxcarbazepine (Trileptal), lamotrigine (Lamictal), levetiracetam (Keppra), toparamate (Topamax), and valproic acid (Valproate). Of all the anticonvulsants, gabapentin has been studied the most extensively for RLS through case series and open-level and limited double-blind studies. It appears to be useful in RLS, particularly in patients who complain of pain. In some RLS patients with pain complaints, pregabalin has also been found to be useful, though extensive studies of this medication have not yet been conducted for this indication. The other anticonvulsants are used rarely in RLS, but may be options for patients who do not respond to gabapentin used in combination with other drugs.

Opioids are painkillers; they are not officially approved by the FDA for RLS, but may offer relief to patients with this condition. The various opioid agents are classified as low-, medium-, and high-potency drugs. Because they are associated with risks of developing addiction, dependence, and tolerance, these medications are not used as first-line drugs for RLS, but rather are reserved for severe and intractable cases, and for patients with augmentation. If an opioid is deemed appropriate, it is best to start with a low-potency drug. If that fails, a medium- or high-potency medication may be prescribed, beginning with a very small dose and gradually increasing the amount of drug taken. Owing to their rapid and short-lasting action, these drugs may also be used on an intermittent, as-needed basis for special situations such as long plane flights, long drives, or watching an evening movie. This practice avoids the risks of tolerance, addiction, and dependence.

Sedative-hypnotics prescribed for RLS include several non-benzodiazepine receptor drugs: zolpidem (Ambien), extended-release zolpidem (Ambien CR), eszopiclone (Lunesta), and zaleplone (Sonata). Ramelteon (Rozerem) is a melatonin receptor agonist used for this disease. Tramadol, a synthetic opioid-like medication, has also been found to be useful for severe RLS symptoms, particularly when symptoms are painful. Sedative-hypnotics are used sparingly and are typically reserved for patients with severe sleep problems associated with RLS symptoms. The benzodiazepine group of drugs has more side effects, including sedation with next-day hangover effects that interfere with daytime function. This side effect may also promote RLS symptoms in the daytime. For treating insomnia in RLS patients, most specialists prescribe non-benzodiazepine drugs and ramelteon because of their shorter half-life, the smaller risk of developing tolerance and dependence, and the less problematic side effects compared to benzodiazepines. It is not a good idea to use these medications every night. Instead, their use should be limited to a few nights each week, with nondrug therapy (e.g., cognitive-behavioral therapy, which includes sleep hygiene measures and relaxation therapy) being used for chronic insomnia.

Therapy should be individualized and is best directed by the physician. Most patients will initially be prescribed a single drug rather than multiple drugs, beginning with a very small dose and gradually increasing the amount taken every five to seven days to an optimal or maximal tolerable dose. Even in an apparently severe case, the physician will begin therapy with a single drug using a small to medium dose. If the patient has been taking multiple drugs for RLS, it is sometimes possible to convert to a single drug by gradually reducing the dosages of some of the other medications. If the patient complains of undesirable side effects from a multidrug treatment, the physician may try to reduce the dose or eliminate some medications. It is very important to have a regular follow-up to monitor for side effects, progression of the disease, augmentation, tolerance, and rebound.

Many patients with mild intermittent RLS will respond to nondrug measures. Unfortunately, these measures may not adequately relieve uncomfortable RLS symptoms in some patients in this group. For these nonresponders,

Many patients with mild intermittent RLS will respond to nondrug measures.

drug treatment may still be needed. It should be noted that RLS medications are approved for moderate and severe RLS, but not for mild RLS cases. Therefore, if patients with mild RLS need medication, dopamine agonists (unapproved for this group) may be tried as the first-line drugs. Alternatively, the physician may prescribe other drugs (e.g., gabapentin or pregabalin) that have not been FDA approved specifically for RLS, but are approved for other diseases—a practice known as "off-label use." (Once a drug is on the market in the United States, physicians can prescribe it for any disease, including conditions for which it was not specifically approved.) According to RLS specialists, if a patient does not respond to one dopamine agonist (i.e., there is a lack of response or problematic side effects occur), then switching to another agonist may be tolerable to the patient. For example, if the patient fails to respond to pramipexole, then he or she may very well respond to ropinirole, and vice versa.

Medications should be taken $1^{1}/_{2}$ to 2 hours before bedtime, as they take time to act. In some patients, an additional dose in the evening to address the evening symptoms may be needed. The physician will always begin by prescribing a very small dose, which will gradually increase every five to seven days. It is best not to exceed the recommended dose, because doing so will increase the chance of severe side effects, including augmentation. If the patient does not respond to a dopamine agonist, then other medications may be tried, either singly or in combination (see Question 80).

72. What are the side effects of dopaminergic and other medications used to treat RLS?

The drugs most commonly used to treat RLS are dopaminergic agents. There is a great individual variation in the occurrence of side effects to these medications. Very common side effects include nausea, dizziness (or faint feelings), sleepiness, and headache. These side effects were found in many of the pivotal drug trials. The drug that has been found to be most helpful to treat nausea is domperidone; this medication is not available in the United States, but can be obtained from Canada or Mexico. The most vexing side effects, particularly during long-term management of RLS, include augmentation, which requires discontinuation in most of these patients (see Questions 73, 74, and 76); tolerance (see Question 75); and rebound (see Question 75). Uncommon side effects of dopaminergic therapy for RLS include impulse control disorders (see Questions 46 and 47), ankle edema (swelling due to fluid collection under the skin), weight gain (see Question 48), and sleepiness and sleep attacks (see Question 77). Other very serious side effects include **fibrosis** (stiffening caused by the buildup of tissue) of the linings of the heart, lungs, and abdomen, giving rise to serious heart, lung, and abdominal diseases, respectively. These complications were noted with ergoline (a compound derived from ergot alkaloids produced by a fungus infecting rye and other plants) dopaminergic agents such as pergolide, which is no longer used because of these side effects. Cabergoline, an ergoline dopaminergic agent with a long duration of action, may have a small chance of causing fibrotic complications; it is not approved for treating RLS, and is very expensive. Other side effects noted with the dopaminergic medications include a reaction to the site where the patch (e.g., rotigotine patch) is applied.

Narcotics or painkillers (opiates or opioids), which are used in severe and refractory cases of RLS and in patients with severe augmentation, commonly cause nausea,

Treatment of Restless Legs Syndrome

Fibrosis

Stiffening caused by the buildup of tissue; scarring.

vomiting, somnolence, lightheadedness, and constipation. More serious side effects include the potential for addiction, dependence, or abuse. Persons with a history of drug abuse in the past should not receive these medications, and they should be monitored for addiction and dependence. Another serious side effect in patients who take large doses of opioids over the long term is respiratory depression, which may cause sleep apnea or worsening of sleep apnea in those who already have the condition. These patients should be carefully monitored using polysomnographic study to detect these adverse respiratory events during sleep.

Side effects of sedative-hypnotic drugs (e.g., benzodiazepine and non-benzodiazepine agonist drugs) include daytime sedation and sleepiness, which may pose a danger for driving and may cause work-related accidents. These medications (particularly benzodiazepines) may also cause addiction, dependence, and respiratory depression, and should be used cautiously in patients with sleep apnea. In fact, these drugs should not be used in patients with sleep apnea unless they are receiving treatment such as continuous positive airway pressure (CPAP) titration.

The anticonvulsant medications that are sometimes used in RLS may cause nausea, dizziness, sleepiness, and next-day adverse effects. Some of these medications may cause more serious side effects such as skin rashes, liver damage, incoordination, and (rarely) bone marrow depression leading to serious depletion of blood cells. Patients taking some of these medications must be monitored regularly and should have regular blood counts and liver function tests performed. Many anticonvulsant medications can produce serious birth defects; thus they should not be used in pregnant patients.

73. I have been taking dopaminergic medication (Sinemet) for my RLS symptoms in the evening and night for more than two years with fairly good response. Lately, my symptoms have begun to start later in the afternoon; they are growing more intense, and sometimes the symptoms spread to my arms. Is this worsening due to the progression of the disease or is it augmentation?

These symptoms are strongly suggestive of augmentation (see Question 74)—the most serious long-term medication-related issue in RLS. The term "augmentation" was introduced by Johns Hopkins investigators in 1996 to describe drug-induced complications of levodopa treatment in RLS patients. Subsequent studies confirmed the features described in the initial report, consisting of earlier onset of symptoms and intensification of symptoms that spread to other body parts. The prevalence of augmentation is noted to be highest with levodopa treatment, but this complication has also been reported with dopamine agonist medications (pramipexole and ropinirole). The lowest risk of augmentation is noted with cabergoline and rotigotine patch treatment for RLS. Most reports of augmentation have described its occurrence with dopaminergic medications, except for two brief reports involving tramadol. Factors influencing the risk of augmentation include the dose of the dopaminergic medication (more chance of augmentation with larger doses), the duration of treatment (more change of augmentation after months of treatment with levodopa), the presence of iron deficiency as measured by serum ferritin (more chance of augmentation in patients with low serum ferritin levels), and the duration of action of the medication (less chance of augmentation with long-duration dopaminergic medications such as cabergoline and rotigotine patch).

74. How is augmentation diagnosed?

Before the National Institutes of Health (NIH)–sponsored RLS workshop in 2002, there were no diagnostic criteria for defining augmentation. Following the workshop, RLS experts developed a set of criteria to diagnose augmentation, which were published in the *Sleep Medicine* journal in 2003. The initial criteria were further refined in an international consensus conference held at the Max Planck Institute in Munich, Germany, and sponsored by the World Association of Sleep Medicine (WASM) and International Restless Legs Syndrome Study Group (IRLSSG). These criteria, which were published in *Sleep Medicine* in 2007, are listed in **Table 10**. The key features supporting a diagnosis of

Table 10   Diagnostic Criteria for Augmentation

A. Prior response to DA medication; an increase of symptom severity on five of seven days for which no other cause

B. A paradoxical response to medication

C. An earlier onset of symptoms by at least 4 hours

   OR

   An earlier onset between 2 and 4 hours

   PLUS

   One of the following:

   • Shorter latency to symptoms when at rest

   • Extension of symptoms to other body parts

   • Greater intensity of symptoms

   • Decreased duration of medication benefit

   Augmentation = A + B; A + C; A + B + C

Source: Garcia-Borreguero D, Allen RP, Kohnen R, et al. Diagnostic standards for dopaminergic augmentation of restless legs syndrome, report from a World Association of Sleep Medicine–International Restless Legs Syndrome Study Group consensus conference at the Max Planck Institute. *Sleep Med* 2007;8:520–530.

augmentation include the following: an earlier onset of symptoms in the evening or afternoon; an increase in the intensity of RLS symptoms, more than the initial baseline symptoms; a shorter latency to onset of symptoms during a period of inactivity; an expansion or spread of symptoms to previously unaffected body parts (e.g., upper limbs, trunk, even genitals and face); and a reduced period of relief following the administration of medication.

75. How is augmentation differentiated from disease progression, tolerance to the drug, or rebound effects of the drugs?

It is sometimes very difficult to differentiate augmentation from symptoms of severe RLS as a result of disease progression. RLS is generally a slowly progressive disease. When the disease progresses to the point that the person has more frequent symptoms with spread of symptoms into the daytime, this stage may be confused with severe augmentation. Cases of augmentation will show a paradoxical response (i.e., on reducing the medication dose, symptoms of augmentation may decrease; on increasing the dose, symptoms may continue to progress). In disease progression, however, any reduction of medication will make the symptoms worse rather than better.

Another important point to differentiate between disease progression and augmentation is that disease progression is generally slow, rather than sudden and acute, except for exacerbation triggered by certain factors (e.g., associated iron deficiency, comorbid medical conditions, ingestion of antidepressants, use of over-the-counter medications such as antihistamines and antinausea drugs, and relatively inactive lifestyle). In contrast, in augmentation, the progression of symptoms could be dramatic, with symptoms suddenly worsening. In other cases, augmentation may present with slowly increasing worsening of the symptoms with fluctuation of symptoms and spread to other body parts.

Rebound is the end of the dose effect, which occurs mainly with medications of short duration of effect such as levodopa. It generally does not occur with dopamine agonists, whose action lasts for 6 to 8 hours. With rebound, the blood level of the medication falls in the early hours of the morning (e.g., 3 to 4 A.M.) accompanied by a resurgence of symptoms. In contrast, augmentation occurs early in the evening or afternoon but not in the early morning. In rebound, after initial exacerbation, there will be symptom-free periods later in the morning. Conversely, symptoms persist in augmentation and may expand to other body parts—a phenomenon that does not occur in rebound. In rebound, there is also no intensification of RLS symptoms.

Tolerance is defined as a decreased response to medication over time requiring an increasing medication dose to achieve the same effectiveness (i.e., an increased need for medication). In the course of time, the effect of dopaminergic agents wears off due to decreased sensitivity of dopamine receptors. The patient thus requires increasing doses of dopaminergic medication to relieve the symptoms. Tolerance does not shift the timing of the symptoms and does not cause more severe symptoms than occurred before starting treatment. In contrast, augmentation is characterized by increasing severity of symptoms, and the severity exceeds the pretreatment severity level. Some investigators think that augmentation goes through a stage of tolerance. A final point to note is that tolerance does not cause the spread of RLS symptoms to other body parts.

Rebound

The end of the dose effect of a medication, in which falling levels of the drug in the body lead to a resurgence of symptoms.

With rebound, the blood level of the medication falls in the early hours of the morning (e.g., 3 to 4 A.M.) accompanied by a resurgence of symptoms.

Tolerance

A decreased response to medication over time, requiring an increasing medication dose to achieve the same effectiveness.

76. How is augmentation treated?

Treatment of augmentation requires the expertise of an RLS specialist. In the absence of a full understanding of the mechanism underlying augmentation, treatment is simply based on expert opinion. The first step is to make a diagnosis of augmentation. The next step is to consider ways to prevent augmentation. Factors that worsen RLS symptoms (see Questions 51, 73, 81, and 82) should first be excluded. If any iron deficiency is noted or if serum ferritin is low, initial treatment should consist of oral iron supplements, along with oral vitamin C to promote iron absorption.

As a preventive measure, a very low dose of dopaminergic medication should be used, with this dose being increased very slowly. Levodopa—the dopaminergic agent most likely to cause augmentation—is generally not prescribed nowadays by specialists to treat RLS because of this tendency. If a patient is treated with levodopa, very small doses should be given. Levodopa, however, can be used intermittently under certain situations (e.g., watching a movie in the theater, listening to a concert, going for a long car ride or plane trip). The advantage of using levodopa under these circumstances is that its action is very quick (within 15 to 30 minutes) and does not last too long; if this drug is used intermittently, the chances of augmentation are minimal.

If symptoms of augmentation are mild and occur in the early afternoon, or if the patient can manage the symptoms by nondrug treatment (e.g., walking and moving around), then there is no need to change the drug regimen. If symptoms are interfering with daytime functioning, then in a mild case, the best strategy is to either split the medication into two doses (one in the early afternoon and one at nighttime, taken 2 hours before bedtime) or add a small dose of dopamine agonist in the afternoon. If the patient continues to exhibit symptoms suggestive of increasing augmentation, a different strategy must be used. Sometimes changing from one agonist to the other—for example, changing from pramipexole to roprinirole, or from roprinirole to pramipexole—may take care of the problem, as there is generally no cross tolerance.

In severe cases of augmentation with more severe restlessness and severe sleep disturbance, this strategy will not work. In such a situation, the dopaminergic medication should be gradually decreased with a view toward stopping it altogether. During this period, the patient may experience severe symptoms lasting for three to four days. The other way to handle this situation is to gradually decrease the dopaminergic medication and simultaneously add another medication, such as a medium-potency opioid or an anticonvulsant (e.g., gabapentin or pregabalin). In very severe cases, high-potency opioids may be given after stopping the dopaminergic medications completely. Sometimes combinations of medications, such as opioids and anticonvulsants (pregabalin or gabapentin), may have to be used. Other measures that may be useful include drug holidays and rotation of drugs (see Question 83).

77. I am an RLS patient on dopaminergic medication. I have had several episodes of sudden attacks of sleepiness in the daytime in an inappropriate time and under inappropriate circumstances. Are these due to medication or RLS?

Sudden attacks of sleepiness in the daytime are not very common in RLS patients, but have been noted in many patients with Parkinson's disease who required much larger doses of dopaminergic medication than those used for RLS. In Parkinson's disease, excessive sleepiness or attacks of sleepiness are most likely due to a combination of the medication (i.e., side effects) and the Parkinson's disease itself, which causes loss of dopaminergic neurons in the brain. In RLS, there is no loss of dopaminergic neurons in the brain and the doses of medication used are relatively small. As a consequence, the likelihood of excessive sleepiness or sleep attacks is rare.

Despite sleep dysfunction, most of the RLS patients do not complain of excessive sleepiness. In fact, they are more likely to report being hyperaroused or hyperalert during the daytime. The cause of this curious phenomenon—that is, sleep deprivation at night and a hyperalert state in the daytime—in many RLS patients is not known.

In one questionnaire survey including 156 RLS patients and 126 control subjects without RLS, a slightly higher prevalence of sudden onset of sleep in RLS patients than in controls was found. This condition was especially pronounced in elderly RLS patients with reduced duration of night sleep. Nevertheless, there is no association between sleepiness and duration or severity of the disease. It is interesting to note that this sleepiness was noted in untreated RLS patients; following dopaminergic treatment, there is a lower risk of sleepiness than occurs in untreated patients. Some anecdotal reports describe RLS patients complaining of sleepiness shortly after starting dopaminergic medication.

On the one hand, most of the reports of daytime sleepiness and sudden sleepiness in RLS patients are probably

Despite sleep dysfunction, most of the RLS patients do not complain of excessive sleepiness.

related to the disease—namely, the severe sleep disturbance at night—rather than to use of dopaminergic
medications. On the other hand, non-dopaminergic
medications, such as sedative-hypnotics (clonazepam),
anticonvulsants (gabapentin or pregabalin), and opiate
medications used to treat severe cases of those with augmentation, may cause daytime sleepiness.

78. I suffer from RLS symptoms intermittently, but the symptoms are intense on some nights. I get these symptoms one or two nights per week. At other times, I remain symptom free for weeks at a time. Should I see my family physician for treatment or should I try over-the-counter medications?

Before you decide on any course of treatment, either
prescribed by your family physician or purchased in
the form of over-the-counter medications, you must be
absolutely certain your symptoms are consistent with a
diagnosis of RLS. You should not make the diagnosis
yourself based on knowledge gathered from the Internet or reading material. If you suspect that you are
experiencing RLS symptoms, you should see your
family physician, provided he or she is knowledgeable
about RLS, or, even better, seek out an RLS specialist
to have the diagnosis confirmed. Once the diagnosis is
established, you have to decide whether you need drug
treatment or whether you can control your symptoms
by nondrug measures as outlined in Question 70.

From the description given in the question, it appears
that the patient goes into remission for weeks and suffers from symptoms only one or two nights per week,
though these symptoms can be intense on occasions.
This patient should try nonpharmacologic measures

first. Under no circumstances should any patient use over-the-counter medications to treat RLS, as many of these medications contain histamines and will aggravate RLS symptoms (see Question 82). If the non-pharmacologic measures do not relieve the symptoms and the symptoms continue interfering with sleep, the patient should see an RLS specialist for treatment.

79. What can I do for my sleep problem associated with my RLS symptoms? Should I take sleeping medications in addition to RLS drugs?

As discussed in Question 27, RLS is associated with significant chronic sleep disruption at night, which may result in serious consequences in both the short and long runs. Many times after satisfactory treatment and relief of RLS symptoms, patients are able to maintain sleep and have adequate hours of sleep at night; these individuals do not need any further treatment for sleep disturbance.

Some RLS patients, however, continue to have problems falling asleep despite satisfactory resolution of the RLS symptoms. Adequate studies (including PSG studies) have not been performed in this group of patients to fully elucidate the nature of their sleep problems. It appears that after being conditioned for months and years by not being able to fall asleep and maintain sleep as a result of RLS symptoms, they are left with persistent insomnia, which requires treatment to ensure optimal functioning during the daytime. Treatment for these patients should follow the principles applied to patients with chronic insomnia. Sleeping medications are generally prescribed for short-term insomnia. In contrast, nondrug therapy, with or without intermittent use of sleeping medications, is the mainstay of treatment for chronic insomnia. A specialist can advise you about appropriate treatment.

Two classes of medications have been approved by regulatory agencies for treating insomnia: benzodiazepine receptor agonists and non-benzodiazepine receptor agonists. Since non-benzodiazepine receptor agonists have become available during the last several years (i.e., zolpidem [Ambien], extended-release zolpidem [Ambien-CR], eszopiclone [Lunesta], zaleplan [Sonata]), these drugs have been used in preference to benzodiazepine receptor agonists because they offer a better side-effect profile. In particular, fewer day-after hangover effects are noted with the non-benzodiazepine agents. Two of the non-benzodiazepine receptor drugs (eszopiclone and extended-release zolpidem) have been found in double-blind, placebo-controlled clinical trials to be relatively safe for use as long as six months. The FDA has also approved a non-benzodiazepine hypnotic for use in patients with sleep-onset insomnia—namely, ramelteon (Rozerem), a melatonin receptor agonist that promotes sleep induction.

If you are taking a sleeping medication, you must be prepared to go to bed immediately after taking the medication and must prepare to have a full night's sleep without getting up and engaging in other activities after taking these medications. If you do not follow these recommendations, there may be serious adverse effects such as sleep walking, confusional arousals, and falls—partial arousals may trigger all of these events. You should not also take a dose higher than the recommended amounts prescribed by your physician.

Nonpharmacologic (nondrug) treatment includes sleep hygiene measures (see Question 70), relaxation therapy, stimulus control therapy, sleep restriction, and patient education about sleep habits and attitude toward sleep (cognitive-behavioral therapy). Relaxation therapy includes progressive muscle relaxation and biofeedback to reduce the arousing stimuli. Stimulus control therapy is directed at discouraging the learned association between the bedroom and wakefulness and at reestablishing the bedroom as the major stimulus for sleep. As part of this therapy, the patient is advised to go to bed when sleepy; not to watch television, eat, or worry while in bed; to use the bed only for sleep; and, if unable to fall asleep within 20 minutes, to get out of bed, go into another room, do something relaxing (such as listening to music or reading light books), and then go back to bed when sleepy. These steps can be repeated. Other recommendations are to wake up at a fixed time each morning, including weekends, and to not take naps.

Cognitive-behavioral therapy (CBT) addresses dysfunctional beliefs and attitudes about sleep. It educates the patient about realistic views regarding the nature of sleep and alleviates any misconceptions the patient may have about sleep. For example, many individuals are under the impression that if they do not have 8 hours of sleep, they cannot function the next day and the short sleeping period will be a disaster for them. This is not true. Each individual's requirement for sleep is different, and the recommended $7^1/_2$ to 8 hours of sleep is just an average figure. Many people can get by with 6 hours or less; others require more than 8 hours of sleep. The important point to emphasize is how the individual functions the next day. If a person can function adequately with sufficient energy and motivation, even if he or she did not have 8 hours of sleep, there is no cause for concern. Similarly, if the patient woke up in the middle of the night and then went back to sleep

Each individual's requirement for sleep is different, and the recommended $7^1/_2$ to 8 hours of sleep is just an average figure.

again quickly, that is acceptable as long as there is no impairment of next-day function.

80. I am a 60-year-old woman and have suffered from RLS for almost all of my life. Medications controlled the symptoms until recently. Now the symptoms are intense and intolerable; they are disturbing my sleep and making my life miserable. Do I have intractable or refractory RLS? How do physicians treat this severe condition?

The situation described here is consistent with very severe or refractory RLS. **Intractable** actually means that the disease is not treatable; **refractory** means it is very difficult to treat.

Intractable

Not treatable (in regard to disease).

Refractory

Difficult to treat (in regard to disease).

RLS specialists define the severity of RLS in various ways (e.g., intermittent, daily, moderate to moderately severe, and refractory RLS). Patients with intermittent or mild RLS complain of symptoms occasionally, and they have long periods of remissions. The majority of these patients do not seek treatment, although some are bothered by the symptoms and need treatment. These patients often respond to nondrug treatment (see Question 70). These patients may need medication on an "as needed" basis in certain situations—for example, during a long plane or car ride, while watching a movie in a theater or listening to a concert. In this situation, the patient may be treated with levodopa (using a very small dose), a low-potency opioid (using a small dose), or one of the first-line drugs such as pramipexole or ropinirole (which should be taken $1^{1}/_{2}$ to 2 hours before the actual situation). All of these treatments must be prescribed by a physician. On the IRLS rating scale (see Question 32), these patients score from 1 to 10.

Patients with moderate to moderately severe RLS experience symptoms almost daily or at least two to three times per week, disturbing their sleep. Their IRLS scores vary from 11 to 20. These patients should use nondrug measures but will also need drug treatment (see Question 71). Most of them respond to FDA-approved dopamine agonist medications. If you have this type of disease, you should follow the recommendations of your physician, who will prescribe medication according to the principles of treatment outlined in Question 71 (i.e., start with a low dose and gradually increase it every 5 to 7 days). An alternative therapy in some of these patients may be off-label use of drugs such as gabapentin or pregabalin at night. The physician will discuss all of these measures with you and recommend the appropriate regimen for your unique situation.

Patients with severe RLS complain of symptoms daily; their IRLS scores vary from 21 to 30. Most of these patients will improve on pramipexole or ropinirole. If the patient does not improve on pramipexole, then the other approved dopamine agonist (ropinirole) should be tried, and vice versa. If a patient cannot tolerate these medications because of their side effects, then alternative drugs such as gabapentin, pregabalin, or opioids (low to medium potency) should be tried on an off-label basis. If needed, these patients can be given high-potency opioids for relief of symptoms.

Refractory patients have RLS scores ranging from 30 to 40 (usually closer to 40). They have severe symptoms every night. These patients usually initially responded to one of the approved dopaminergic medications but over the course of time, the response became inadequate. In another group of patients, the initial response may have been inadequate despite taking an adequate dose. These patients need increasing doses of medication to obtain relief. In these individuals, the possibility of augmentation must be considered and ruled out (see Question 74). The physician should also consider and rule out triggering factors such as lifestyle situations (sedentary habits), use of other medications (see Question 81), and comorbid conditions.

In patients with refractory RLS, the dose of the initial medication should be gradually increased, but the maximum recommended dose should not be exceeded to avoid unacceptable adverse effects. There are no standard guidelines in this scenario; rather, the treatment is based on expert opinion. In this situation, the physician will likely prescribe one or more drugs on an off-label basis. Anticonvulsants (gabapentin, pregabalin, or others), medium- to high-potency opioids, or a combination of these off-label drugs and dopaminergic medications (which are specifically approved for use in RLS) in some cases may work. Some patients with refractory disease will respond to drug holidays or drug rotations (see Question 83). If all medications fail to relieve the symptoms, there is no alternative except to use high-potency opioids such as methadone. This treatment of last resort must be carefully monitored by the physician.

Elda's comment:

"Can't you ever sit still?" I hated when the teacher would yell at me. I was only about 12 years old. I just couldn't contain the energy that seemed to be ready to explode in my feet and lower legs. Continually moving them, swinging them, stamping them was the only thing that helped, but only momentarily. I had pains in my legs at night, which my mother called growing pains, but the feelings of about-to-explode energy only happened during the day. This continued on through several years of high school, but around age 17 or so, stopped.

Fast forward to around age 40 ...

I started to get feelings of intense heat in my feet at night, burning so badly I remember walking barefooted on the snow just to cool them off, or standing in a tub in cold water. Even when visiting friends in Canada, I remember walking out in the deep snow, trying to anesthetize the burning in my feet. Gradually, the feelings of burning changed into feelings of either the about-to-explode energy, or bugs, maggots, moving around in the soles of my feet. As the years passed, these feelings became more and more frequent, and the feeling of bugs moving around inside my feet became more and more pronounced. I tried to tell my doctor about it, various doctors actually, but none ever tried to explain it, and none even wrote it down in my medical records. My symptoms were especially maddening during my menstrual period—even later, when I had medications to help me cope, the RLS during menstrual times was just awful.

By age 45 or so, I was feeling quite isolated with these awful feelings that deprived me of relaxation and sleep each and every night. With no doctors to help, I was dealing with this all alone. I reasoned, accurately, it seems, that this was some sort of neurological disorder, so I went on the Internet to find something—anything—that would help. I found an herb, Valerian Root, which was a nerve tonic, so I tried various preparations. I found one brand of Valerian Root (Nature's Way) that actually helped! I'd take one or two capsules at bedtime, and could sleep. The Valerian Root was a godsend for several years, but gradually lost its efficacy. I was back to kicking all night long, walking through the wee hours of the morning. Again, I was asking for my doctors' help in dealing with this condition, but none were able to help. I think they were ready to send me for a psychiatric consultation, since none of them even wrote this down in my medical file, again!

Treatment of Restless Legs Syndrome

It was around this time that two different people came to my assistance. The first was my massage therapist: she noticed how fatigued I was all the time, and when I told her about my continuing problems with this terrible maggoty feeling in my feet, she said she had just read about this in her Massage Therapist's Journal, and that it was called "Restless Legs Syndrome." Eureka! I had a name to work with, something to Google! Around the same time, a work associate came into my office to discuss a project, and during the course of our talk, mentioned that he was constantly being awakened at night by his wife's kicking and jumping and frequent awakenings. He said his wife had Restless Legs Syndrome. But she was not just another patient—his wife was a doctor, a surgeon! I commiserated with him about his inability to get a good night's sleep, but most especially, identified with his wife. I only worked in an office— no big life-and-death stress. Sleepiness for her, however, any mistake, especially during an operation, could be disastrous! It was she who found the NJ Neuroscience Institute (NJ NSI) and she passed this information on to me.

At the Institute, the doctor initially prescribed Neurontin (Gabapentin), which immediately helped. I felt like this terrible weight had been lifted! I could sleep, I could watch TV, go to the movies, or simply just read without constantly kicking, squirming around, stamping my feet, or having to just get up and walk. After about 8 months or so, the Neurontin began to be less effective, so the doctor increased the number of capsules prescribed. This helped for a while, but again and again, the dose had to be increased due to the Neurontin becoming less effective. This was the first time it happened, but a phenomenon called "augmentation" began to happen. As my RLS symptoms continued to worsen, the doctor kept increasing the number of capsules. Then my RLS symptoms started occurring earlier and earlier in the day and lasting later at night and into the early morning hours, until I was experiencing the symptoms from around 2 P.M until perhaps 6 A.M. At that point, I think I was taking 6 or 8 Neurontin capsules a day, 2 every 4 hours starting around 2 P.M. Then something paradoxical happened: the very medication that had stopped the RLS symptoms started to actually cause them! At its worst, instead of just feeling the creepy-crawly feelings in my feet, they expanded to my legs, arms, hands, trunk, and even my vagina. I can honestly say that while I live with chronic pain from Fibromyalgia and Osteoarthritis, the only time in my life I've ever felt suicidal was when experiencing the RLS symptoms vaginally. (Augmentation and tolerance happened not only with Neurontin, but later with Requip and later still, with Ultram, including the expansion of symptoms to arms, hands, trunk, and vagina.) These effects seem to happen for some reason in my physiology with medications that are not usually associated with it.

After I was no longer able to take the Neurontin, the doctor prescribed Requip. After approximately 8 or 9 months, the same scenario unfolded.

I have tried a variety of medications or remedies to help control the RLS symptoms. Finally, the Institute doctors prescribed Methadone to control my RLS symptoms.

I have been taking Methadone with good results ever since. I understand that I am currently taking a great many medications for my physical problems, and am concerned about their effects, side effects, and interactions. The Methadone, especially, concerns me since I am rather fearful of its narcotic effects, so try to be very judicious in its use. I am grateful that it is working and that my Restless Legs Syndrome symptoms are controlled with a relatively small dose.

In June, 2009, my Rheumatologist prescribed a drug called Savella to help with the Fibromyalgia. It was in an ascending dose start-up packet. The initial week's dose was low, and that was fine; although it did not help the Fibromyalgia. When I started Week 2, however, where the dose increased sharply, my Restless Legs Syndrome dramatically increased to the point that I was experiencing it all day and all night. I called the doctor at the Institute and he doubled my Methadone dose. I took the higher dose for several days until the Savella was out of my system, then resumed my regular dose of one Methadone tablet every other night. It seems to have a long half-life, so it alleviates the symptoms for me for more than one night.

I'm grateful to all the doctors at NJ NSI for their knowledge, patience, and wisdom.

81. My RLS specialist told me that certain medications and agents can worsen my RLS symptoms and I should avoid these medications. What are these medications?

Certain types of medications can worsen RLS symptoms: All RLS patients, RLS specialists, and general physicians and others who are likely to take care of RLS patients should be aware of these medications. Although there are no validated scientific studies to prove beyond a shadow of a doubt that these drugs exacerbate the disease, there are sufficient reports from a large number of patients, not only in practice but also in the published literature, about the triggering effects of these medications to warrant avoiding them in patients with RLS. For unknown reasons, a subset of patients do not experience worsening of their RLS symptoms upon ingesting these medications. Given that there is no way of knowing who will and will not have exacerbation of the disease, it is best to avoid these medications in patients with RLS symptoms if at all possible. These medications can be classified into four broad groups: (1) antidepressants,

(2) antihistamines, (3) antinausea drugs, and (4) antipsychotic medications.

Almost all antidepressant medications make RLS symptoms worse through serotonin mechanisms. Both selective serotonin reuptake inhibitors (SSRIs) and selective serotonin and norepinephrine reuptake inhibitors (SSNRIs) are used to treat patients with depression. The SSRIs include citalopram (Celexa), escitalopram (Lexapro), sertraline (Zoloft), fluoxetine (Prozac), and paroxetine (Paxil). The SSNRIs include duloxetine (Cymbalta) and venlafaxine (Effexor). Both types of antidepressants will worsen RLS symptoms in most patients; thus, if possible, their use should be avoided in RLS patients, and alternative antidepressants should be prescribed.

Almost all antidepressant medications make RLS symptoms worse through serotonin mechanisms.

Tricyclic antidepressants (TCAs) were very popular in the past, but have fallen out of favor as treatments for depression in recent years because of their troublesome side effects and because of the availability of newer, better antidepressants. Based on the chemical structure of the compound, TCAs are divided into two groups: tertiary amines, which worsen RLS symptoms through a serotonin mechanism, and secondary amines, which act through the mechanism of mainly norepinephrine and do not worsen RLS symptoms. Examples of tertiary amines include amitriptyline (Elavil), clomipramine (Anafranil), doxipen (Sinequan), and imipramine (Tofranil). Examples of secondary amines include desipramine (Norpramin), nortriptyline (Pamelor), and protriptyline (Vivactil).

Two antidepressants do not aggravate RLS symptoms: bupropion (Welbutrin), which has a dopamine agonist action and may actually improve RLS symptoms, and trazodone (Desyrel). Mirtazapine (Remeron) belongs to a new class of antidepressants and also tends to worsen RLS symptoms.

Treatment of Restless Legs Syndrome

Most of the antihistamines are notorious for exacerbation of RLS symptoms in most of the patients and, therefore, should be avoided if possible. Most over-the-counter sleeping pills contain doxylamine or diphenhydramine (both are antihistamines), so they should not be used as sleeping medications by patients with RLS. Three antihistamine drugs are probably relatively safe in terms of not causing exacerbation of RLS symptoms: Claritin, Clarinex, and Allegra.

Like antihistamines, antinausea drugs tend to exacerbate RLS symptoms because they block the dopamine receptors in the brain. Examples of these drugs include metoclopramide (Raglan), prochlorprazine (Compazine), meclizine (Antivert), hydroxyzine (Atarax), and promethazine (Phenergan). Except for metoclopramide, these drugs can be called the "-zine" group of drugs. Some alternative drugs available to treat nausea do not seem to aggravate RLS symptoms. One of them is domperidone, which is not available in the United States but may be obtained from Canada or Mexico. The three drugs in the "-citron" group of drugs are used to treat severe nausea (and are very expensive), but do not appear to exacerbate RLS: granicitron (Kytril), ondancitron (Zofran), and dolacitron (Anzemet). Another antinausea medication that does not appear to aggravate RLS symptoms is transdermal scopolamine, which is generally used for motion sickness.

The fourth class of drugs that aggravate RLS symptoms includes the antipsychotics (neuroleptics), which are used to treat major psychiatric disorders such as schizophrenia, bipolar disorders, or other psychoses. These dopamine-blocking agents are highly likely to aggravate the RLS symptoms; their opposites, the dopaminergic medications, do help RLS patients. Examples of antipsychotic medications that may exacerbate RLS include haloperidol, clozapine, olanzapine, resperidine (Resperdal), and quetiapin (Seroquel). One newer antipsychotic drug called aripiprazole (Abilify) is a dopamine agonist and does not aggravate RLS symptoms. In fact, many patients report improvement of their RLS symptoms with aripiprazole because of its dopaminergic action.

All RLS patients should routinely discuss their current medications with their physicians. In addition, they should periodically review their medications with all of their physicians to avoid acute exacerbation of their RLS symptoms from this source.

82. I am a 60-year-old man who has severe depression. Recently, my psychiatrist put me on a strong antidepressant medication (a selective serotonin reuptake inhibitor). Soon after I started taking the medication, my RLS symptoms (which I have had for the last 10 years) became worse. They are now intolerable. Should I stop taking the antidepressant?

You should not abruptly stop taking your medication, but rather should consult your psychiatrist and RLS specialist about what you should do. This scenario can sometimes be very difficult to manage. It should be looked at in two different ways: Did the symptoms of severe depression precede the RLS, or did the depression emerge after the diagnosis of RLS? In other words, do you have primary depression *separate from* RLS or do you have depression *as a result of* RLS symptoms?

Epidemiological surveys and case series have confirmed that after suffering from RLS symptoms and insomnia for long periods of time, patients with RLS often develop depression. There is a two-way relationship between insomnia and depression. Someone suffering from insomnia for a long time has a much greater chance of developing depression within 12 months; conversely, someone suffering from depression may develop symptoms of insomnia.

As stated in Question 81, most of the widely used antidepressant medications—which include selective serotonin reuptake inhibitors (SSRIs), selective serotonin and norepinephrine reuptake inhibitors (SSNRIs), and tricyclic antidepressants (TCAs)—will worsen RLS symptoms. There are, of course, exceptions. Unfortunately, the patient described in this question is not in the exception group. If your depression is severe and you are having suicidal thoughts, you must be monitored by your psychiatrist for management with antidepressants. Certain antidepressants do not exacerbate RLS symptoms, such as bupropion and trazodone (see Question 81). It is worth trying these medications first in a patient with RLS before SSRIs are used. If these agents do not relieve the depression, other medications must be used. If the depression is severe and does not respond to any of these medications, the psychiatrist will probably prescribe SSRIs, albeit starting with a small dose.

One strategy in this patient's case might be reducing the SSRI dose and adding a more RLS-friendly antidepressant such as bupropion. The psychiatrist will determine whether this option is appropriate.

If the patient fails to respond to any measures other than SSRIs, then another strategy is to increase the RLS medication to the maximum recommended dose. If this approach does not relieve the RLS symptoms, then the dopaminergic medication can be combined with other RLS drugs (gabapentin or pregabalin, or a benzodiazepine at night). If the RLS symptoms are very severe, intolerable, and making the patient miserable, then the doctor may prescribe medium- to high-potency opioid medications for the RLS and continue the antidepressant medications to control the depression.

The patient in this question has described a very difficult situation, and one that is very difficult to treat. If you are in this situation, you should not despair: Most of the time, it is possible to treat both conditions (depression and RLS) satisfactorily by trial and error with medications. During this treatment, you should avoid other factors that might trigger the RLS (see Question 51) and continue with any nonpharmacologic treatment (see Question 70). Note that all of the suggestions presented here are based on expert opinion—studies of severe RLS associated with severe depression have yet to be undertaken.

83. I read on the Internet that for severe and intractable RLS, sometimes drug holidays and rotating the medications may be useful. I was warned that the information on the Internet may occasionally be misleading and false. What should I do?

You should listen to your physician. In some severe or refractory cases of RLS, as well as those with severe augmentation, drug holidays or rotations of medications may help. Note that there have not been adequate scientific studies to prove the effectiveness of these measures.

The principle underlying **drug holidays** relates to the concept of tolerance (see Question 75). Increasing medication doses may cause receptor desensitization and failure of response. Under these circumstances, drug holidays (i.e., withholding the medications for a few weeks or two

Drug holiday
Withholding use of a medication for a few weeks or two to three months, or taking the medication two to four times per week rather than daily.

to three months) may restore the sensitivity of the receptors after some time. Tolerance to medication may be noticed with dopamine agonists, opioids, and benzodiazepine (clonazepam) drugs. After drug holidays, the medication is restarted with a small dose and increased slowly. An alternative to this kind of drug holiday is taking the medication two to four times per week rather than daily, which is equivalent to a short drug holiday.

Rotation of medication is based on the same principle of tolerance. Rotation of one agonist with another every two to three months may prevent the development of tolerance (there is no cross-tolerance noted with dopamine agonists, but this effect may occur with opioids or benzodiazepines). Opioids or benzodiazepines may also be rotated with other drugs such as anticonvulsants (gabapentin or pregabalin) and dopamine agonists.

Drug holidays and rotation of medications have not been scientifically studied systematically in a large number of patients. Therefore, the value of this modality of treatment is based on anecdotal evidence.

84. I am a 62-year-old woman who is scheduled to have knee replacement surgery. Should I tell my surgeon or my anesthesiologist that I have RLS, or should I keep quiet about my RLS because these physicians may think that all my symptoms are psychosomatic?

You very definitely must tell your surgeon and the anesthesiologist that you have RLS.

You very definitely must tell your surgeon and the anesthesiologist that you have RLS. It is important to do so because many factors during the preoperative and postoperative periods may worsen RLS symptoms, including the anesthetic agents used during surgery. RLS symptoms have been reported to worsen after several types of surgeries—for example, gastric surgery, above-the-knee amputation, and lung surgery. The mechanisms involved are not known, but several factors might contribute to the worsening of RLS symptoms: postoperative or intra-operative prolonged immobilization of the legs, blood loss causing iron deficiency, sleep deprivation in the hospital, and use of a variety of medications including antihistamines and antinausea drugs. In such a case, existing RLS symptoms may become worse or RLS symptoms may appear for the first time in those persons who are genetically predisposed to have RLS.

The medications used to control RLS may have to be increased temporarily before and after surgery. In the immediate postoperative period, generally opioids are given to control the pain which will also help RLS. As their effects wear off, symptoms will reemerge. For this reason, it is very important for all patients with RLS to inform the surgeon and anesthesiologist about their condition before surgery.

Interestingly, RLS symptoms may improve or disappear after certain surgeries—for example, kidney transplantation in patients with RLS associated with kidney failure. There is one report of improvement of comorbid RLS symptoms in a patient with Parkinson's disease after surgical intervention involving the basal ganglia.

85. My Chinese girlfriend told me that I should try acupuncture and herbal medications for my RLS symptoms. Should I listen to her advice or should I see an RLS specialist?

There is no proof that acupuncture or herbal medications relieve RLS symptoms. Acupuncture is sometimes used for pain and discomfort when all else fails, out of sheer despair and frustration. Some anecdotal reports describe improvement of RLS symptoms after acupuncture, but there are no double-blind, validated studies to prove the effectiveness of acupuncture except for some limited studies in Chinese traditional medicine journals published in China.

Similarly, herbal medications are often advertised as "magic" cures for all sorts of diseases, including RLS, and are readily available in health food stores and via the Internet. These medicines are frequently used by RLS patients, but with contradictory results—either temporary relief or no relief at all. Again, there is no valid study to prove the effectiveness of the herbal medications.

The author of this book does not recommend herbal medications or acupuncture for patients with RLS symptoms causing discomfort and disturbing sleep. Instead, patients should consult their physicians, who will recommend the appropriate therapy for them.

86. Is there a role for complementary and alternative medicine in the treatment of RLS?

Complementary and alternative medicine (CAM)

Non-allopathic medicine, including non-conventional medicine, mind–body interactions, naturopathy, manipulative therapy, and electromagnetic therapy.

Complementary and alternative medicine (CAM) includes a variety of nonconventional measures used by specialties other than allopathic (conventional) medicine. These measures may include exercises, meditations, foods, and others that are thought to be helpful in all bodily and mental illnesses, including RLS. CAM options can be classified into five categories: nonconventional medicine, mind–body interactions, naturopathy, manipulative therapy, and electromagnetic therapy (see **Table 11**).

There are many anecdotal reports of benefits from complementary and alternative medicine in a variety of illnesses, including RLS. You can readily find an enormous amount of advertisement on the Internet promoting

Table 11   Complementary and Alternative Medicine

Nonconventional Medicine (i.e., other than allopathic medicine)
- Homeopathic medicine (as practiced in India and other countries)
- Ayurvedic medicine (practiced in India) using natural plants and seeds
- Naturopathic medicine
- Traditional Chinese medicine (TCM)

Mind–Body Interaction
- Meditation
- Prayer
- Yoga
- Creative therapies to control body functions (e.g., art, music, dance)

Naturopathy
- Herbs
- Special foods
- Vitamins

Manipulative Therapy
- Osteopathy
- Chiropractic care

Electromagnetic Therapy
- Magnets

CAM therapies for all varieties of illnesses. The problem is that no validated scientific studies have been undertaken to prove the efficacy of these measures on a lasting basis. In many patients, including RLS patients, CAM therapy often gives temporary relief through the "placebo effect" (see Question 94).

Because of many reports (including some scattered case reports) showing possible benefit from CAM therapy in RLS and other illnesses, the National Institutes of Health (NIH) recently created the National Center for Complementary and Alternative Medicine (NCCAM, www.nccam.nih.gov). This site is designed to serve as a clearinghouse for validated information on CAM therapies.

Treatment of Restless Legs Syndrome

A word of caution is in order, however: Many CAM therapies interact with other medications, sometimes causing adverse effects. Furthermore, the long-term effects of many of these CAM therapies are unknown. Without evidence from rigorous scientific studies, it is not advisable to use CAM therapies to treat RLS, even out of utter frustration and helplessness (which RLS patients sometimes suffer). The best advice is to discuss with your physician the role of CAM therapy before using any such therapy on your own.

The only exceptions to this recommendation are meditation, relaxation, yoga, and other kinds of relaxing exercises. These measures may promote good sleep and, therefore, are recommended to those RLS patients who are left with persistent sleep problems despite getting adequate relief of their RLS symptoms from traditional medications.

87. I read that taking lots of vitamins and minerals will cure my RLS and I do not need any prescription medications. Is this true?

There are no scientific studies to prove, one way or the other, what role vitamins or minerals play in RLS. Periodically, RLS patients claim benefits from taking vitamin A, B, C, D, or E; folic acid; calcium; magnesium; zinc; fish oil; or other supplements. Advertisers take advantage of these anecdotal reports to promote their products. Some limited studies show benefit for patients who take vitamin B_{12}, folic acid, and magnesium. Nevertheless, without large-scale placebo-controlled studies, the significance of these findings remains controversial. The only thing we know definitely is that iron is beneficial in some RLS patients with low iron in the body and the brain, as documented by low ferritin levels in the blood and cerebrospinal fluid.

88. Are there any preventive measures I can take before prolonged sedentary periods (e.g., going to a movie, show, or concert; going on a long plane or car ride; having an MRI test requiring the need to lie down quietly inside the scanning machine)?

You can definitely take some preventive measures to prevent emergence of RLS symptoms during these sedentary situations. The decision about which measures are appropriate should be made in consultation with your physician. For example, you can take a low- to medium-potency opioid, which will act quickly within 15 to 20 minutes and produce effects that last for 2 to 3 hours without causing any long-term undesirable effects. Similarly, you can take a small dose of levodopa; because it acts quickly and the duration of its effect is short, this usage will not lead to augmentation or other long-term side effects of levodopa. You can also take your regular approved dopamine medication if you are using one for RLS symptoms. You must take this medication at least $1^1/_2$ to 2 hours before the situation in which you need temporary relief, because both pramipexole and ropinirole (the standard recommended dopaminergic medications) take time to reach effective levels in the blood).

89. I have heard that patients with severe Parkinson's disease are treated with deep brain stimulation. Given that both RLS and Parkinson's disease result from dopamine dysfunction, can deep brain stimulation also be a treatment for intractable or refractory RLS?

Deep brain stimulation (DBS)—that is, stimulating certain parts of the basal ganglia or thalamus—has

Deep brain stimulation (DBS)

Stimulation of certain parts of the basal ganglia or thalamus. This technique is occasionally used as a treatment for severe Parkinson's disease.

been used in some severe cases of Parkinson's disease (i.e., in patients who failed to respond to the standard treatment) with good relief of symptoms. As yet, there are only isolated case reports of its use in RLS patients. In one report, DBS stimulation in Parkinson's disease improved comorbid RLS symptoms. In another report, DBS stimulation of thalamus for essential tremor improved the tremor but did not improve the comorbid RLS symptoms. Hence, with only contradictory isolated case reports and without an adequate validated study in a large number of patients, this question remains unanswered at the present time. Furthermore, in contrast to Parkinson's disease, RLS patients do not have loss of nerve cells in the basal ganglia, which calls into question the rationale for use of DBS in RLS.

90. How do physicians treat periodic limb movements in sleep and periodic limb movement disorder? At what point in the disease course does this treatment begin?

Actual treatment should be tailored by a physician. To fully address this question, it is necessary to discuss the controversy regarding periodic limb movements in sleep (PLMS) and **periodic limb movement disorder (PLMD)**. PLMS has been noted in about 80% of patients with RLS but has also been noted in some primary sleep disorders such as **narcolepsy** (an illness characterized by uncontrollable or excessive sleepiness under inappropriate circumstances and during inappropriate times, either with or without sudden loss of muscle tone, and occurring during periods of emotional excitement such as laughter, fear, or anger), **rapid eye movement sleep behavior disorder** (a condition characterized by dream-enacting behavior, mostly about frightening events occurring during the dream stage

Periodic limb movement disorder (PLMD)

A disorder characterized by the presence of periodic limb movements in sleep, causing insomnia or hypersomnia symptoms.

Narcolepsy

An illness characterized by uncontrollable or excessive sleepiness under inappropriate circumstances and during inappropriate times, either with or without sudden loss of muscle tone, and occurring during periods of emotional excitement such as laughter, fear, or anger.

Rapid eye movement (REM) sleep behavior disorder

A condition characterized by dream-enacting behavior, mostly about frightening events occurring during the dream stage of sleep.

of sleep), and **obstructive sleep apnea syndrome** (a condition characterized by daytime sleepiness, snoring and repeated cessation of breathing during sleep associated with short-term and long-term adverse consequences leading to high blood pressure, stroke, heart attacks, and memory impairment). In addition to these conditions, PLMS has been noted after use of certain medications and in many normal individuals, particularly in normal elderly people.

Because of its presence in a variety of conditions, including in normal individuals, many sleep specialists believe that PLMS is simply a polysomnographic finding that causes no particular sleep-related symptoms. In contrast, other sleep specialists believe that PLMS is a sleep disturbance giving rise to insomnia or excessive daytime sleepiness. In fact, the International Classification of Sleep Disorders lists PLMD as an entity characterized by the presence of PLMS causing insomnia or hypersomnia symptoms. The problem is that there have not been scientifically validated studies proving that PLMS can occur alone, without any associated comorbid conditions such as RLS, narcolepsy, REM behavior disorder, obstructive sleep apnea syndrome, or other conditions that cause insomnia or daytime sleepiness. Recently, it has been shown that PLMS is accompanied by increased heart rate and rise of blood pressure transiently. If these effects happen repeatedly, long-term PLMS may eventually cause sustained high blood pressure or may be responsible for cardiovascular disorders. There is no scientifically validated proof for this hypothesis. Therefore, if your physician is convinced that PLMS causes symptoms, then PLMS should be treated.

On many occasions, it is the bed partner—rather than the patient—who complains about the patient's leg

---

Obstructive sleep apnea syndrome (OSAS)

A condition characterized by daytime sleepiness, snoring and repeated cessation of breathing during sleep associated with short-term and long-term adverse consequences leading to high blood pressure, stroke, heart attacks, and memory impairment.

Treatment of Restless Legs Syndrome

jerking. In such a case, all parties involved must decide whether it is appropriate to treat the patient just to satisfy the bed partner or whether other measures (such as using separate beds for the bed partners) are appropriate, given that treating the patient with medication may have harmful side effects.

After considering all of these issues, if the decision is made to treat the patient, then the best and first-line treatment will be those dopaminergic medications (pramipexole or ropinirole) approved for RLS treatment, beginning with a very small dose and increasing the dose very slowly. An alternative treatment is to use gabapentin or pregabalin (at least in some patients). Finally, some physicians have treated RLS patients with benzodiazepines or benzodiazepine receptor agonists; these medications probably do not decrease PLMS, but decrease repeated arousals associated with PLMS and promote sleep onset and sleep maintenance, thereby giving symptomatic relief.

91. I am a 60-year-old woman who has been taking opioids for severe and intractable RLS for two years. Recently, I have been feeling very fatigued during the daytime, and my bed partner noticed that my breathing has been irregular, with pauses in breathing during sleep. What is happening to me?

Opioids (a group of synthetic morphine drugs) may be prescribed in very severe and refractory RLS cases.

Opioids
A group of synthetic morphine drugs.

Opioids (a group of synthetic morphine drugs) may be prescribed in very severe and refractory RLS cases. The best way to treat such severe disease is to use, if possible, low- to medium-potency opioids rather than high-potency opioids, and to use the smallest dose needed to obtain relief.

Opioids and other morphine derivatives have a direct depressing effect on the nerve cells in the brain stem that control breathing. In patients on long-term opioid medications, there is a real danger of breathing being affected, leading to periodic or irregular breathing with impairment of breathing effort and air flow through the nose and mouth. The only way to confirm this problem is by doing a polysomnographic study. Nevertheless, there should be a high index of clinical suspicion, which can be addressed by monitoring the patient, asking about the daytime symptoms of sleepiness and fatigue, and asking the bed partner about witnessed apneas.

A PSG study may document abnormal breathing patterns, which will require treatment. The first step in treatment is to consider decreasing or discontinuing opioids and replacing them with other suitable medications. The abnormal breathing should be treated by upper airway pressurization using bilevel positive airway pressure or assisted servo ventilation with or without supplemental oxygen administration during sleep at night. Your physician will be the best person to advise you regarding the treatment. The most important point is that the patients on long-term opioids should be monitored on a regular basis by polysomnographic study to detect abnormal breathing patterns that may have been caused by the medications.

92. A friend who has RLS received Botox injections for RLS symptoms and obtained some relief. What is Botox injection and does it help RLS?

Botulinum toxin A (brand name: Botox), when injected intramuscularly, causes temporary paralysis of neuromuscular junctions (the junctions of the nerve and muscle where the nerve impulses stimulate receptors to create an electric current, which in turn stimulates the muscle to act). This treatment has been used effectively in many patients with certain movement disorders (e.g., some local or segmental hyperactivity of the muscle of unknown cause). Recently, it has been used for cosmetic purposes, for which Botox is injected under the skin to stretch the skin and temporarily remove creases. There are isolated case reports—but no validated studies—indicating that Botox injections may relieve RLS symptoms.

93. Are there any new medications undergoing clinical trials that may be available soon? What are the advantages of these new medications?

The search for an ideal drug for RLS goes on. The currently approved first-line medications—the dopaminergic drugs (pramipexole and ropinirole)—relieve the symptoms in most patients, at least in the beginning of the disease course, but are associated with some short-term and many long-term adverse consequences. One of the most troublesome of these complications is augmentation, which typically makes patients stop these dopaminergic medications after months or years of symptomatic relief.

Because of these vexing side effects, several new medications are undergoing clinical trials. One is a dopaminergic medication named rotigotine that is available in a patch form; this method of administering the drug ensures 24-hour continuous delivery of the active ingredient, without any pulsatile variations in the amount delivered. It is hoped that this medication will decrease the chances of augmentation. The rotigotine patch is now approved for treating Parkinson's disease but has not yet been approved for RLS patients. Trials using this medication are continuing, and the FDA may soon approve this drug for treating RLS symptoms.

XP13512, a gabapentin prodrug (gabapentin enacarbil), has undergone some clinical trials with satisfactory results in RLS patients. Gabapentin has been found to be useful in many RLS patients, not only in open-level clinical trials, but also in double-blind, placebo-controlled clinical trials. There is, however, considerable individual variation in terms of its effectiveness. Specifically, gabapentin's efficacy is affected by factors such as the variable rate of absorption and the drug's absorption through only a limited region of the small intestine (the portion of the gut largely responsible for absorption of nutrients from food as well as many medications). XP13512 is well absorbed throughout the entire length of the small intestine. On absorption, it is rapidly converted to gabapentin. In contrast to gabapentin, whose rate of absorption declines with increasing dose, XP13512 shows dose-proportional absorption and superior bioavailability, and it produces a more predictable response. Several trials have shown good response in RLS patients to this compound, but the FDA has not yet approved the drug for use in the general population.

Another anticonvulsant, pregabalin, has been found to be effective (in off-label use) in several RLS patients (anecdotal evidence), and limited studies have shown its effectiveness in this population. This drug appears to be promising, but placebo-controlled clinical trials need to be performed in a large number of RLS patients before the efficacy of this drug can be stated with authority and an application can be filed with the FDA for approval of its use in RLS.

The advantages of some of the new medications—for example, pregabalin and XP13512—are that these drugs belong to a class of medications different from the dopaminergic agents. For this reason, it is assumed that these medications will not cause the troublesome side effect of augmentation and will lead to sustained relief of RLS symptoms. In the future, other classes of medications may be tried in RLS patients that might open up opportunities for additional treatments and better understanding of the pathophysiology of RLS.

94. In clinical drug trials focusing on RLS, some patients get a placebo and some get the real drug. What is a placebo and why is it used?

The word "placebo" in Latin means "I shall please." A **placebo** is a fake (sham) medical intervention. It is used in most clinical trials, although patients are not told that it is not the real medicine. The patients in most clinical trials are told that some subjects will be given inert ("sugar") pills that will look exactly like the real pill and that some subjects will be given the real medicine. Both the subjects and the investigators may remain "blind" to which subjects receive the real treatment and the placebo, in which case the trial is called a "double-blind," placebo-controlled clinical trial. This design is the preferred way of studying the effectiveness of a medication.

Placebo

A fake (sham) medical intervention.

The subjects receiving the placebo are known as the control group; the others are labeled as the treatment group. Some patients who receive placebo, believing that they are receiving the real medication, get a "therapeutic" benefit from the "treatment." This psychological benefit may last for some time, but eventually the symptoms reappear.

Placebos are widely used in clinical drug trials. The success of a placebo in relieving symptoms, even though this effect is temporary, speaks strongly about the mind–body relationship. The mechanism by which the placebo effect occurs is not known. It has been found that RLS patients are particularly susceptible to the placebo effect, and a large percentage of RLS subjects given placebo get temporary relief from their symptoms. Why RLS patients are more susceptible than other patients to the placebo effect is not known. It is possible that a predisposition to both development of RLS symptoms and response to placebo may be responsible for this phenomenon in RLS patients.

PART SIX

Coping and Management Techniques

What is the role of exercise and lifestyle
changes in treatment of RLS?

What is the role of nutrients and certain foods
in RLS treatment?

How do physicians treat RLS in children?

More . . .

95. How does one cope with a condition such as RLS that is often misdiagnosed, misunderstood, and labeled as a psychosomatic (psychoneurotic) disorder?

RLS is a chronic progressive disorder with considerable morbidity that affects quality of life, alters relationships with family and friends, and interferes with lifestyle and other pleasures of life. On top of all this, the condition frequently goes undiagnosed or is underdiagnosed. Even today, some patients with RLS are misdiagnosed and thought to be suffering from psychosomatic disorders.

These misunderstandings place a tremendous burden on patients with RLS. Perhaps not surprisingly, some of these individuals also have anxiety and depression. Under these circumstances, it is sometimes very difficult to cope with all of these adverse features. Nevertheless, there are many coping strategies that patients can adopt and should follow.

First and foremost is to obtain education and knowledge about the condition. Patients with RLS should recognize that they must schedule their activities in such a way that they are not immobile for prolonged periods of time—after all, RLS is a disease of quiescence. Lifestyles may need to be modified as well. For example, persons with RLS should stop smoking and drinking alcohol, and should avoid consuming caffeinated beverages, as all of these practices may impact RLS symptoms adversely. Affected individuals should also follow the recommended sleep hygiene practices (see Question 70).

Patients should avoid, as much as possible, all RLS triggers and the medications and agents that are known to worsen RLS symptoms (see Questions 51 and 81).

Patients should consume nutritious and balanced diets and engage in regular moderate exercise, while avoiding excessively strenuous exercise. Measures that can relieve RLS symptoms include mental and physical activities, mental distraction, counter-stimulation measures, and, in some patients, sexual activity. Patients should avoid, as much as possible, anger and frustration; they should also resist the urge to eat and drink in the middle of the night. Patients should take preventive measures during certain special situations such as long plane trips and long drives. Many patients suffer from depression and anxiety, which should be addressed appropriately. Finally, it is important to join RLS support groups to listen to other people; participating in such groups can minimize the frustration and loneliness that many people with RLS feel. All of these coping strategies have been found to be helpful in many RLS sufferers.

Patients should consume nutritious and balanced diets and engage in regular moderate exercise, while avoiding excessively strenuous exercise.

96. What is the role of exercise and lifestyle changes in treatment of RLS?

Exercise in moderation has been found to be helpful in most of the RLS patients, although no randomized, controlled trials have been conducted to prove this point. Overly strenuous exercise may aggravate RLS symptoms. Physical activities such as walking, stretching, rubbing, and massaging can often relieve RLS symptoms successfully, without drug treatment, in mild to moderate cases of RLS. Exercise should be avoided too close to bedtime, as physical exercise increases body temperature and stimulates arousal mechanisms, thereby preventing sleep. A falling body temperature is conducive to sleep; hence exercise approximately 5 to 6 hours before bedtime is best for initiation of sleep. Exercise also is thought to promote sleep efficiency, increase sleep duration, and encourage sleep onset. A sedentary lifestyle will aggravate RLS symptoms, as RLS is a disease of quiescence. Other lifestyle features that may be cited as triggers for RLS include smoking and increasing body weight (see Question 48). A change of lifestyle (e.g., semi-retirement, relatively inactive lifestyle) may cause a sudden exacerbation of RLS.

97. What is the role of nutrients and certain foods in RLS treatment?

Adequate nutrition and balanced diet are important in most diseases, including RLS. Whether some particular diet helps alleviate RLS symptoms remains controversial. There are anecdotal reports of worsening RLS symptoms after eating ice cream and improvement after reducing consumption of carbohydrates and wheat (which contains gluten). If you have celiac disease and RLS, reducing your consumption of gluten (white flour) will be helpful (see Question 60). There are no scientific studies to prove that a particular diet or a nutrient either improves or worsens RLS symptoms. Conversely, it is well known that smoking, consuming alcohol, and drinking caffeinated beverages aggravate RLS symptoms in most patients.

98. I am in my third trimester of pregnancy and my RLS symptoms are getting worse, seriously affecting my quality of life. My obstetrical/gynecological specialist told me to avoid all medications, as they may harm the baby. What should I do?

Pregnancy is a risk factor for RLS. Both new-onset RLS symptoms and aggravation of ongoing RLS symptoms have been noted in 20 to 25% of pregnant women (see Question 9). The symptoms are particularly severe during the third trimester, but rapidly disappear or dramatically decrease in intensity and frequency shortly after delivery of the baby, regardless of treatment.

Treatment of RLS symptoms during pregnancy is a challenge for physicians because of the possible harmful effects of medications to the unborn baby, including teratogenecity. It is best to avoid any medications if possible and rely on nonpharmacologic treatment in such cases (see Question 70). Patients with mild to moderate RLS may be able to cope with these symptoms by using nondrug therapy. It is important to measure serum iron, ferritin, folate, and magnesium levels in the pregnant woman with RLS. If a subnormal level is found, supplementation may be recommended; however, there is no guarantee that such treatment will improve or relieve RLS symptoms. In severe cases, if RLS symptoms remain intolerable despite nonpharmacologic measures, causing severe sleep disturbance and impairing quality of life, drug treatment may be needed.

For purposes of determining the safety of medications to the fetus, the FDA has classified drugs into five categories. Category A is safe without known harmful effects to the fetus: There are no category A RLS drugs available. Categories B, C, and D represent increasingly unsafe drugs for the fetus, and Category X includes drugs that are considered unsafe and contraindicated in pregnancy. Category B includes cabergoline, pergolide, low-dose methadone, and short-term use of oxycodone. Category C includes the RLS-approved dopaminergic drugs (e.g., pramipexole and ropinirole) as well as the anticonvulsants. Category D includes benzodiazepines, high-dose methadone, and long-term use of oxycodone. Thus the only drugs that could be used during pregnancy with mild risk to the fetus are low-dose methadone and short-term oxycodone. The pregnant woman should consult with her obstetrical/gynecological specialist before taking any of these medications. It is also advisable to discuss with the pediatrician any possible danger from these medications to the fetus.

Most medications used to treat RLS, including opioids, are secreted in breast milk and, therefore, may pass to the newborn child through breastfeeding. For this reason, it is best not to breastfeed while taking these medications. Nursing mothers should not be given dopamine agonists, as these drugs decrease prolactin, which will in turn decrease production of breast milk. Ideally, opioids should not be used during late pregnancy because of possible respiratory depression to the newborn or withdrawal syndrome.

99. How do physicians treat RLS in children?

There are no American Academy of Sleep Medicine (AASM) or European Federation of Neurological Society (EFNS) guidelines for drug treatment of RLS in children, as there is insufficient evidence to support long-term efficacy of drug treatment in childhood RLS. The first-line therapy consists of nonpharmacologic measures (see Question 70) similar to those used for treating adult RLS patients. Serum iron and ferritin levels should be measured in children with RLS; if these levels are found to be low, iron therapy should be given to the child. Nondrug treatment includes good sleep hygiene measures and avoiding sleep deprivation; avoiding medications that might aggravate RLS such as antihistamines and antinausea drugs; and avoiding caffeinated beverages and foods containing chocolate. There are only limited reports of treatment of children with dopaminergic medications (e.g., pramipexole and ropinirole), but these drugs are used on an off-label basis in pediatric patients (i.e., the FDA has not approved their use in children). The dose administered to children should be less than that used in adults, and pediatric patients should be maintained on these drugs at a minimum dose. Treatment should be monitored under the close supervision of a pediatric specialist with experience and knowledge in RLS or a sleep specialist with experience in pediatric medicine.

100. Where can I get more information about RLS?

Please turn to the Resources appendix at the end of the book for more information about the organizations and resources available for those suffering from RLS.

Coping and Management Techniques

Resources

You can obtain essential information about restless legs syndrome (RLS) from a number of professional and lay organizations. A number of Web sites also disseminate valuable information about RLS directed specifically to the public; this information has been written by doctors. In addition, many books are devoted to RLS. The sources listed here should point you in the right direction.

American Academy of Sleep Medicine (AASM)
2510 North Frontage Road
Darien, IL 60561
Telephone: 708-492-0930
www.aasm.org
The mission of the AASM is to promote sleep disorders medicine to members
  of the medical and paramedical professions as well as to the public. The
  organization is dedicated to supporting quality care for patients with sleep
  disorders, providing professional and public education on the issues, and
  encouraging and supporting research in sleep medicine.

National Center for Sleep Disorders Research (NCSDR)
2 Rockledge Center, Suite 7024
6701 Rockledge Drive, MSC7920
Bethesda, MD 20892-7920
Telephone: 301-435-0199
www.nhlbi.nih.gov/sleep
The NCSDR was established after a national commission on sleep disorders
  research, which was mandated by Congress, recommended in 1993 that a
  national center for research and education in sleep and sleep disorders be
  established. This center is located within the National Heart, Lung, and
  Blood Institute of the National Institutes of Health (NIH) in Bethesda,
  Maryland. It supports research, education, and training in sleep and sleep
  disorders for all healthcare professionals. The center also participates in public
  awareness and education campaigns about sleep disorders. It works in
  collaboration with several federal agencies, including the NIH; the former

Alcohol, Drug Abuse, and Mental Health Administrations; and the Departments of Defense, Transportation, and Veterans Affairs.

National Sleep Foundation (NSF)
729 Fifteenth Street, NW, 4th Floor
Washington, DC 20005
Telephone: 202-347-3471
www.sleepfoundation.org
The NSF produces valuable brochures dealing with sleep and sleep disorders, promotes public education (particularly about driving, fatigue, and sleepiness as well as important sleep disorders), and periodically organizes Gallup polls dealing with sleep and sleep difficulties.

Restless Legs Syndrome (RLS) Foundation
1610 14th Street, NW, Suite 300
Rochester, MN 55901
Telephone: 507-287-6465
www.rls.org
The RLS Foundation was established by patients suffering from RLS in 1990 and is guided by an RLS scientific advisory board and a medical advisory board. Its mission is to support patients with RLS and their families. The RLS Foundation also provides information to educate health care providers about RLS and sponsors research intended to find better treatments and, eventually, a definitive cure. Members (patients with RLS) receive newsletters with valuable information about the disease and support groups throughout the country.

Recommended Books on Restless Legs Syndrome

Buchfuhrer MJ, Hening WA, Kushida CA (eds). *Restless legs syndrome: Coping with your sleepless nights.* New York, Demos Medical Publishing, 2006.

Chaudhuri KR, Odin P, Olanow CW. *Restless legs syndrome.* New York, Taylor and Francis, 2004.

Gunzel J. *Restless legs syndrome: The RLS rebel's survival guide.* Tucson, AZ, Wheatmark, 2006.

Hening WA, Allen RP, Chokroverty S, Earley CJ. *Restless legs syndrome.* Philadelphia, PA, Saunders/Elsevier, 2009.

Hening WA, Buchfuhrer MJ, Lee HB. *Clinical management of restless legs syndrome.* West Islip, NY, Professional Communications, 2008.

The official patient's source book on restless legs syndrome. San Diego, CA, Icon Health Publications, 2002.

Ondo WG. *Restless legs syndrome: Neurological disease and therapy.* New York, Informa Healthcare/Taylor and Francis, 2006.

Wilson VA, Walters AS (eds). *Sleep thief: Restless legs syndrome.* Orange Park, FL, Galaxy Books, 1996.

Yoakum R. *Restless legs syndrome: Relief and hope for sleepless victims of a hidden epidemic.* New York, Simon and Schuster, 2006.

Recommended Journals for RLS publications

Sleep Medicine. This international journal is affiliated with the World Association of Sleep Medicine, an international organization for sleep clinicians. It has published most of the important articles dealing with RLS.

Sleep. This journal is affiliated with the American Academy of Sleep Medicine and the Sleep Research Society. It has published many major articles in RLS.

Journal of Sleep Research. This is the affiliated journal of the European Sleep Research Society and has published several important articles on RLS.

Appendix

Actigraphy: A test in which a motion detector is placed on the leg, and leg movements are monitored to assess periodic leg movements in sleep (PLMS).

Adenoids: Lymphoid tissues in the throat behind the nasal passage.

Akathisia: A "subjective desire to be in constant motion" associated with "an inability to sit or stand still" and a "drive to pace up and down" [FDA definition].

Attention-deficit/hyperactivity disorder (ADHD): A disorder characterized by fidgetiness, excessive motor restlessness, inattention, and (in some patients) impulsivity.

Augmentation: Drug-induced complications first noted with levodopa treatment, consisting of earlier onset of symptoms and intensification of symptoms that spread to other body parts.

Autonomic nervous system: The part of the nervous system responsible for controlling involuntary functions such as blood circulation and respiration.

Basal ganglia: Groups of nerve cells and connecting fibers and neurons located deep in the brain that control movements, gait, posture, and emotions.

Brain stem: The lower part of the brain, which is connected to the main portion of the brain and controls vital functions such as circulation, respiration, and sleep.

Central nervous system (CNS): The brain and the spinal cord.

Cerebral hemisphere: The main part of the brain. The right cerebral hemisphere controls the left side of the body; the left cerebral hemisphere controls the right side of the body.

Cerebrospinal fluid: The fluid bathing the brain and the spinal cord.

Chronic fatigue syndrome (CFS): A complex and debilitating illness in which patients complain of profound fatigue that is not improved by bed rest.

Chronic obstructive pulmonary disease (COPD): Chronic bronchitis and emphysema.

Circadian: Occurring in a roughly 24-hour cycle.

Comorbid: Coexisting.

Complementary and alternative medicine (CAM): Non-allopathic medicine, including nonconventional medicine, mind–body interactions, naturopathy, manipulative therapy, and electromagnetic therapy.

Deep brain stimulation (DBS): Stimulation of certain parts of the basal ganglia or thalamus. This technique is occasionally used as a treatment for severe Parkinson's disease.

Diabetes mellitus: A condition in which a person has a high glucose (blood sugar) level, either because the body fails to produce enough insulin or because the cells do not properly respond to the insulin that is produced.

Diaphragm: The main muscle of breathing, separating the lower chest from the upper abdomen.

Dopamine: A neurotransmitter made in the nerve cells that helps transmit nerve impulses to other nerve cells.

Drug holiday: Withholding use of a medication for a few weeks or two to three months, or taking the medication two to four times per week rather than daily.

Electrocardiogram (ECG): A recording of the heart rhythm.

Electroencephalogram (EEG): A recording of the electrical activity of the brain.

Electromyogram (EMG): A recording of the electrical activity of the muscles.

Electro-oculogram (EOG): A recording of the electrical activity associated with eye movements.

False positive: A result that appears to be positive (indicating the presence of disease) when it is actually normal (no disease).

Ferritin: A protein in the blood that is responsible for systemic iron storage; it binds to iron in the blood.

Fibromyalgia: A type of rheumatic disease that does not affect the bones or joints; characterized by diffuse muscle aches and pains throughout the body.

Fibrosis: Stiffening caused by the buildup of tissue; scarring.

Habit spasms: Repetitive limb movements that are performed voluntarily initially, but later become habits.

Hyperalgesia: Excessive perception of pain.

Hypnic jerks: A normal physiological phenomenon characterized by sudden jerking movements of the legs and the whole body that last for a few seconds and always occur at the moment of falling asleep.

Hypopnea: A sleep disorder in which breathing may not stop completely but rather is reduced by 30 to 50% of the normal breathing volume.

Hypothalamus: A group of nerve cells and fibers located in the deeper part of the brain that serves as a center for controlling secretion of hormones, food and water intake, and sleep–wake regulation.

Idiopathic case: A case not associated with other diseases and for which no cause is found.

Impulse control disorders (ICDs): Compulsive behaviors such as compulsive gambling, smoking, eating, punding, or sexual behavior.

Incidence: The number of new cases in a given population during a stated period.

International RLS Study Group Rating Scale (IRLS): The most widely used scale for identifying the severity of RLS; it measures the magnitude of RLS symptoms as well as the impact of symptoms on sleep, daytime function, and mood.

Intractable: Not treatable (in regard to disease).

Kidneys: The pair of organs that is responsible for urine production and excretion from the body.

Limbic cortex: The emotional brain; it plays a central role in perception of pain.

Lungs: The breathing organs responsible for maintaining normal respiration and blood oxygen at the optimal level.

Melatonin: A hormone secreted by the pineal gland in the deeper part of the center of the brain at night, which serves as a circadian marker.

Morbidity: Illness of health.

Narcolepsy: An illness characterized by uncontrollable or excessive sleepiness under inappropriate circumstances and during inappropriate times, either with or without sudden loss of muscle tone, and occurring during periods of emotional excitement such as laughter, fear, or anger.

Narcotics: Central analgesic (pain relief) medications.

Neuroleptic: Nerve-calming medication.

Neuromodulators: Chemicals in the brain that cause activation of the synapses of the nerve cell responsible for pain perception, memory storage, and sleep–wake regulation.

Neuropathy: Damage to peripheral nerves.

Neurotransmitters: Chemicals responsible for transmitting nerve signals.

Nocturnal eating/drinking syndrome: A sleep disorder in which a person wakes up repeatedly during the night to eat and drink and has insomnia, but is fully alert during the episode and can recall it the next morning.

Obstructive sleep apnea syndrome (OSAS): A condition characterized by daytime sleepiness, snoring and repeated cessation of breathing during sleep associated with short-term and long-term adverse consequences leading to high blood pressure, stroke, heart attacks, and memory impairment.

Opioids: A group of synthetic morphine drugs.

Parkinson's disease: A degenerative disorder of the central nervous system that often impairs the sufferer's motor skills, speech, and posture.

Periodic limb movement disorder (PLMD): A disorder characterized by the presence of periodic limb movements in sleep, causing insomnia or hypersomnia symptoms.

Periodic limb movements in sleep (PLMS): Leg movements that occur periodically during sleep and that are present in at least 80% of RLS.

Periodic limb movements in wakefulness (PLMW): Leg movements that occur periodically during relative inactivity and that are characteristic of RLS.

Peripheral nervous system: The part of the nervous system that lies outside the central nervous system.

Placebo: A fake (sham) medical intervention.

Polysomnographic (PSG) study: A recording of activities (physiological characteristics) from many body systems and organs during sleep at night.

Prevalence: The number of cases of a disease, whether old or new, existing within a given population at a stated point in time.

Punding: Complex, repetitive, purposeless behaviors.

Quiescence: Being still or inactive; being at rest.

Rapid eye movement (REM) sleep behavior disorder: A condition characterized by dream-enacting behavior, mostly about frightening events occurring during the dream stage of sleep.

Rebound: The end of the dose effect of a medication, in which falling levels of the drug in the body lead to a resurgence of symptoms.

Refractory: Difficult to treat (in regard to disease).

Restless legs syndrome (RLS): A sensorimotor neurologic and movement disorder that seriously affects sleep and quality of life.

Sensorimotor neuropathies: Nerve dysfunction causing sensory symptoms such as tingling and numbness and motor disturbances such as muscle weakness.

Sleep apnea: Cessation of breathing occurring during sleep.

Sleep-related eating disorder: A sleep disorder in which a person has recurrent episodes of eating and drinking during partial arousals from slow-wave sleep.

Soft palate: A soft muscular tissue in the back of the roof of the mouth.

Spinal cord: The long tubular structure of the central nervous system that connects to the brain stem and runs through the vertebral column.

Suggested immobilization test (SIT): A test in which the patient sits quietly with legs outstretched, and leg movements are monitored to assess periodic leg movements in wakefulness (PLMW).

"Sundowning" syndrome (nighttime agitation syndrome): A condition associated with Alzheimer's disease in which the sleep–wake cycle is reversed so that the person is active and agitated at night and sleepy throughout the day.

Thalamus: The main structure in the base of the brain responsible for termination of the ascending pain and other sensory fibers.

Tolerance: A decreased response to medication over time, requiring an increasing medication dose to achieve the same effectiveness.

Uvula: The small piece of soft pear-shaped structure that can be seen dangling down from the soft palate from the back of the tongue.

Index

Index

Index

FORSYTH COUNTY PUBLIC
LIBRARY

Forsyth County Public Library
585 Dahlonega Road
Cumming, GA 30040
www.forsythpl.org

Contact Us:
770-781-9840

Renewals:
770-781-9865